Revisional Foot and Ankle Surgery

Guest Editor

JEROME K. STECK, DPM, FACFAS

CLINICS IN PODIATRIC MEDICINE AND SURGERY

www.podiatric.theclinics.com

Consulting Editor

THOMAS ZGONIS, DPM, FACFAS

January 2009 • Volume 26 • Number 1

SAUNDERS an imprint of ELSEVIER, Inc.

W.B. SAUNDERS COMPANY
A Division of Elsevier Inc.

1600 John F. Kennedy Boulevard • Suite 1800 • Philadelphia, Pennsylvania 19103-2899

http://www.theclinics.com

CLINICS IN PODIATRIC MEDICINE AND SURGERY Volume 26, Number 1
January 2009 ISSN 0891-8422, ISBN-13: 978-1-4377-0530-0, ISBN-10: 1-4377-0530-8

Editor: Patrick Manley
Developmental Editor: Donald Mumford

Clinics in Podiatric Medicine and Surgery (ISSN 0891-8422) is published quarterly by Elsevier Inc., 360 Park Avenue South, New York, NY 10010-1710. Months of publication are January, April, July, and October. Business and Editorial Offices: 1600 John F. Kennedy Blvd., Suite 1800, Philadelphia, PA 191023-2899. Customer Service Office: 6277 Sea Harbor Drive, Orlando, FL 32887-4800. Periodicals postage paid at New York, NY, and additional mailing offices. Subscription prices are $229.00 per year for US individuals, $360.00 per year for US institutions, $118.00 per year for US students and residents, $275.00 per year for Canadian individuals, $445.00 for Canadian institutions, $326.00 for international individuals, $445.00 per year for international institutions and $167.00 per year for Canadian and foreign students/residents. To receive student/resident rate, orders must be accompanied by name of affiliated institution, date of term, and the *signature* of program/residency coordinator on institution letterhead. Orders will be billed at individual rate until proof of status is received. Foreign air speed delivery is included in all *Clinics* subscription prices. All prices are subject to change without notice. POSTMASTER: Send address changes to *Clinics in Podiatric Medicine and Surgery*, Elsevier Periodicals Customer Service, 6277 Sea Harbor Drive, Orlando, FL 32887-4800. **Customer Service: 1-800-654-2452 (US). From outside of the US, call 314-453-7041. Fax: 314-453-5170. E-mail: JournalsCustomerService-usa@elsevier.com (for print support); JournalsOnlineSupport-usa@elsevier.com (for online support).**

Reprints. For copies of 100 or more of articles in this publication, please contact the Commercial Reprints Department, Elsevier Inc., 360 Park Avenue South, New York, NY 10010-1710. Tel.: 212-633-3812; Fax: 212-462-1935; E-mail: reprints@elsevier.com.

Clinics in Podiatric Medicine and Surgery is covered in *MEDLINE/PubMed (Index Medicus) and EMBASE/Excerpta Medica.*

Printed and bound by CPI Group (UK) Ltd, Croydon, CR0 4YY

Transferred to Digital Print 2011

Contributors

CONSULTING EDITOR

THOMAS ZGONIS, DPM, FACFAS
Associate Professor, Department of Orthopaedics; Chief, Division of Podiatric Medicine and Surgery; Director, Reconstructive Foot and Ankle Fellowship, The University of Texas Health Science Center at San Antonio, San Antonio, Texas

GUEST EDITOR

JEROME K. STECK, DPM, FACFAS
Southern Arizona Orthopaedics, Assistant Clinical Professor of Surgery, University of Arizona, Tucson, Arizona

AUTHORS

ESTHER S. BARNES, DPM
Resident, Highlands - Presbyterian/St. Luke's Podiatric Medicine and Surgery Residency Program, Denver, Colorado

RONALD BELCZYK, DPM, AACFAS
Fellow, Reconstructive Foot and Ankle Surgery, and Clinical Instructor, Division of Podiatric Medicine and Surgery, Department of Orthopaedics, The University of Texas Health Science Center at San Antonio, San Antonio, Texas

DAMIEON BROWN, DPM
Fellow, Reconstructive Rearfoot and Ankle Surgical Fellowship, Ohio College of Podiatric Medicine, Ankle and Foot Care Centers, Youngstown, Ohio

JARRETT D. CAIN, DPM, MSc, AACFAS
Podiatric Foot and Ankle Surgeon, West Jersey Health System, Camden, New Jersey

ALAN R. CATANZARITI, DPM, FACFAS
Director of Residency Training, Department of Foot and Ankle Surgery, The Western Pennsylvania Hospital, Pittsburgh, Pennsylvania

RICHARD DERNER, DPM, FACFAS
Private practice, Associated Foot and Ankle Centers of Northern Virginia, Lake Ridge, Virginia

LAWRENCE A. DIDOMENICO, DPM, FACFAS
Director, Reconstructive Rearfoot and Ankle Surgical Fellowship, and Adjunct Professor, Ohio College of Podiatric Medicine, Ankle and Foot Care Centers, Youngstown, Ohio

KRIS DINUCCI, DPM, FACFAS
Podiatric Foot and Ankle Surgeon, Foot and Ankle Center of Arizona, Scottsdale, Arizona

GRAHAM A. HAMILTON, DPM, FACFAS
Department of Orthopedics, Kaiser Foundation Hospital, Antioch, California

LUKE C. JEFFRIES, DPM, AACFAS
Former Reconstructive Foot and Ankle Surgery Fellow and Clinical Instructor, Division of Podiatric Medicine and Surgery, Department of Orthopaedic Surgery, The University of Texas Health Science Center at San Antonio, San Antonio, Texas

MEAGAN JENNINGS, DPM, AACFAS
Department of Orthopedics, Palo Alto Foundation Medical Foundation, Camino Division, Mountain View, California

MICHAEL S. LEE, DPM, FACFAS
Associate Clinical Professor, College of Podiatric Medicine and Surgery, Des Moines University, Des Moines; Private practice, Central Iowa Orthopaedics, Des Moines, Iowa

JARED M. MAKER, BS
Third-Year Student, College of Podiatric Medicine and Surgery, Des Moines University, Des Moines, Iowa

OTTONIEL MEJIA, DPM
University of California Los Angeles Podiatry Group, Los Angeles, California

ROBERT W. MENDICINO, DPM, FACFAS
Chair, Department of Foot and Ankle Surgery, The Western Pennsylvania Hospital, Pittsburgh, Pennsylvania

ANDREW J. MEYR, DPM
Resident, INOVA Fairfax Hospital Podiatric Surgical Residency Program, INOVA Fairfax Hospital, Falls Church, Virginia

LARA J. MURPHY, DPM
Third Year and Chief Resident, Department of Foot and Ankle Surgery, The Western Pennsylvania Hospital, Pittsburgh, Pennsylvania

ALAN NG, DPM, FACFAS
Attending Physician, Highlands - Presbyterian/St. Luke's Podiatric Medicine and Surgery Residency Program, Denver, Colorado

ROBERTO H. RODRIGUEZ, DPM, AACFAS
Assistant Professor, Division of Podiatric Medicine and Surgery, Department of Orthopaedic Surgery, The University of Texas Health Science Center at San Antonio, San Antonio, Texas

THOMAS S. ROUKIS, DPM, PhD, FACFAS
Chief, Limb Preservation Service and Director, Limb Preservation Complex Lower Extremity Surgery and Research Fellowship, Limb Preservation Service, Vascular/Endovascular Surgery Service, Department of Surgery, Madigan Army Medical Center, MCHJ-SV, Tacoma, Washington

SHANNON M. RUSH, DPM, FACFAS
Department of Orthopedics, Palo Alto Foundation Medical Foundation, Camino Division, Mountain View, California

MONICA H. SCHWEINBERGER, DPM, AACFAS
Former Fellow, Limb Preservation Complex Lower Extremity Surgery and Research Fellowship, Limb Preservation Service, Vascular/Endovascular Surgery Service, Department of Surgery, Madigan Army Medical Center, MCHJ-SV, Tacoma, Washington

JOHN J. STAPLETON, DPM, AACFAS
Associate, Foot and Ankle Surgery, VSAS Orthopaedics, Allentown; and Clinical Assistant Professor of Surgery, Penn State College of Medicine, Hershey, Pennsylvania

GLENN M. WEINRAUB, DPM, FACFAS
Kaiser Permanente Medical Group, Department of Orthopaedic Surgery, Hayward/Fremont, California

THOMAS ZGONIS, DPM, FACFAS
Associate Professor, Department of Orthopaedics; Chief, Division of Podiatric Medicine and Surgery; Director, Reconstructive Foot and Ankle Fellowship, The University of Texas Health Science Center at San Antonio, San Antonio, Texas

Contents

Foreword xv

Thomas Zgonis

Preface xvii

Jerome K. Steck

Wound Complications 1

Monica H. Schweinberger and Thomas S. Roukis

This article discusses postoperative wound complications in detail, including host factors that predispose the patient to nonhealing, technical factors in surgery that can reduce the likelihood of infection and dehiscence, and recommendations for postoperative management that can prevent wound healing problems. This discussion includes the treatment of wound complications, ranging from local wound care to various wound coverage options.

Revisional Peripheral Nerve Surgery 11

Jarrett D. Cain and Kris DiNucci

Peripheral nerve disorders are difficult to manage. In the surgical treatment of patients with peripheral nerve pathology, there are a multitude of factors that may alter the outcome of the patient's recovery and lead to incomplete recovery or possibly worsening of symptoms. The anatomy and function of the peripheral nerve is unique and the evaluation and management of these disorders must be approached in a manner different from musculoskeletal disorders. Many anatomic areas can tolerate scar tissue and adhesions, but in peripheral nerves, loss of the gliding functional and adherence to surrounding soft tissue structures is a common complication from over-zealous dissection and repeat peripheral nerve surgery without modification of technique. The approach to each patient must be thorough and individualized to treat their specific condition, and the surgeon must be aware that at times, the most appropriate treatment for the patient may not be medical but surgical management of the chronic pain condition.

Revisional Charcot Foot and Ankle Surgery 127

John J. Stapleton, Ronald Belczyk, and Thomas Zgonis

Charcot neuroarthropathy is often a devastating diabetic foot complication that poses a great risk for limb loss and can have a significant impact on a patient's quality of life in the presence of multiple existing comorbidities. It is a progressive and debilitating condition characterized by joint dislocation, pathologic fracture(s), and extensive destruction of the foot or ankle architecture secondary to dense peripheral neuropathy. This pathologic process can be idiopathic, secondary to acute trauma or previous surgery, or attributable to repetitive "microinjury." Once the Charcot process has been initiated, continued ambulation results in progressive collapse and deformity. Severe deformities can have an impact on the patient's ambulatory status, and when associated with instability, ulceration, or infection, there is greater risk for a major limb amputation.

Current Concepts and Techniques in Foot and Ankle Surgery

The Use of Ilizarov Technique as a Definitive Percutaneous Reduction for Ankle Fractures in Patients Who Have Diabetes Mellitus and Peripheral Vascular Disease 141

Lawrence A. DiDomenico, Damieon Brown, and Thomas Zgonis

The patient who has a diagnosis of diabetes mellitus, diabetic peripheral neuropathy, peripheral vascular disease and experiences an unstable ankle fracture presents as a difficult case scenario for the treating physician. In addition, patients who have diabetes mellitus, along with the presence of multiple comorbidities, have been shown to have higher complication rates than patients who do not have diabetes mellitus. This article describes a relatively safe alternative rgical percutaneous technique using external circular ring fixation in the vascularly compromised diabetic patient with an unstable ankle fracture. This novel technique decreases the risk for soft tissue complications in the high-risk diabetic patient and serves as a definitive method of fixation without the need for additional surgery. It allows the patient to have early and full weight bearing when indicated in the postoperative period.

Pan–Metatarsophalangeal Joint Arthrodesis for the Severe Rheumatoid Forefoot Deformity 149

Luke C. Jeffries, Roberto H. Rodriguez, John J. Stapleton, and Thomas Zgonis

The standard approach for correction of severe painful rheumatoid forefoot deformities has involved resection of the metatarsal heads with realignment of the lesser toe deformities and first metatarsophalangeal joint (MTPJ) arthrodesis. Modifications of this procedure may include a pan–metatarsal head resection, including the first metatarsal head, or resection of the lesser metatarsal heads in conjunction with an interpositional arthroplasty of the first MTPJ. The authors describe a novel surgical approach that involves the correction of severe rheumatoid forefoot deformities through a pan-MTPJ arthrodesis. Arthrodesis of all five MTPJs for the surgical treatment of the painful rheumatoid forefoot deformity with chronic plantar callosities and dislocated digits has yet to be reported in the scientific literature. The goal of this article is to provide the treating physician with another alternative and safe surgical approach when dealing with the painful rheumatoid forefoot deformity.

Index **159**

FORTHCOMING ISSUES

April 2009
Update on Ankle Arthritis
Alan Catanzariti, DPM and
Robert Mendicino, DPM,
Guest Editors

July 2009
The Importance of the First Ray
Lawrence Ford, DPM, *Guest Editor*

October 2009
Advances in Wound and Bone Healing
Adam S. Landsman, DPM, *Guest Editor*

RECENT ISSUES

October 2008
Surgical Reconstruction of the High-Risk Patient
Thomas S. Roukis, DPM, PhD, FACFAS,
Guest Editor

July 2008
Pain Management
Andrew J. Meyr, DPM and
John S. Steinberg, DPM,
Guest Editors

April 2008
Imaging
Denise M. Mandi, DPM,
Guest Editor

RELATED INTEREST

Foot and Ankle Clinics
Volume 13, Issue 4, Pages 571–800 (December 2008)
Current Management of Foot and Ankle Trauma
Edited by M.P. Clare

Foreword

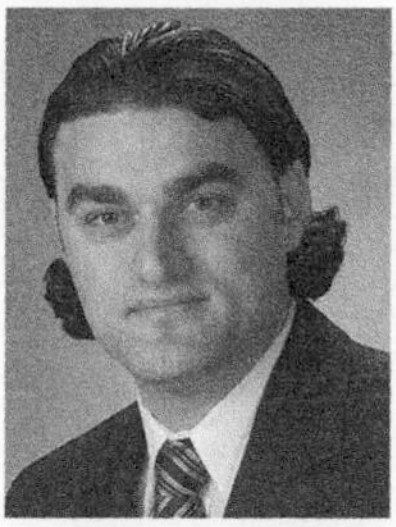

Thomas Zgonis, DPM, FACFAS
Consulting Editor

The greatest fear every surgeon has to face is the possibility of postoperative complications. The fear of the unknown, especially dealing with the prediction of surgical outcome, is the most difficult to conquer. How often do we think twice before a minor or major surgical procedure regarding precautions to take to minimize the possibility of postoperative complications? What preoperative teaching and explanation do we offer our patients before the surgical procedure(s) and how do we cope with their preoperative questions and concerns about the proposed surgery?

I am a strong believer that preventing or at least minimizing postoperative complications starts during the preoperative visit(s) and initial assessments. Explaining to the patient in the presence of a witness all of the conservative and surgical treatment options is a must, and needs to happen with each and every patient before surgery. Also necessary to discuss before surgery are the preoperative laboratory testing, medical imaging, medical clearance and all services used in treatment of the patient's pre-existing conditions. A detailed consent form including all possible minor and major postoperative complications must be signed by a witness before the surgery as well. In addition, the surgeon must explain the possibility of a revisional surgery in the event of postoperative complications, and avoid offering any certain guarantees in response to very high patient expectations.

Revisional foot and ankle cases are even more difficult secondary to inherent conditions such as scar contractures and soft tissue compromise, non-healing incisions, disuse osteopenia, nonunion and/or malunion, deep infection, and failed fixation. Neglecting issues such as patient compliance and psychosocial challenges will only lead to further complications regardless of the surgical plan. Thorough communication with the patient's family members and/or the previous treating physicians needs to be carried out before the revisional surgery is performed.

In this issue, Dr. Steck and his colleagues have done an outstanding job in gathering and presenting some of the most difficult revisional foot and ankle surgery cases. I hope that this issue will become a great tool and also provide great guidance for

Clin Podiatr Med Surg 26 (2009) xv–xvi
doi:10.1016/j.cpm.2008.12.001

your revisional surgical procedures. Lastly, I want to thank the guest editor and invited authors, as well as the editorial board members for their continuous support and contribution to *Clinics in Podiatric Medicine and Surgery.*

Thomas Zgonis, DPM, FACFAS
Associate Professor, Department of Orthopaedics
Chief, Division of Podiatric Medicine and Surgery
The University of Texas Health Science Center at San Antonio
7703 Floyd Curl Drive – MSC 7776
San Antonio, TX 78229, USA

E-mail address:
zgonis@uthscsa.edu

Preface

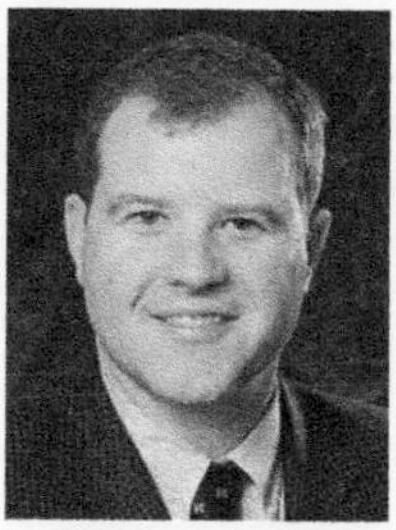

Jerome K. Steck, DPM, FACFAS
Guest Editor

I know of no more encouraging fact than the unquestioned ability of a man to elevate his life by conscious endeavor.

—Henry David Thoreau

It is an honor to be the guest editor for this issue of *Clinics in Podiatric Medicine and Surgery*. Revisional foot and ankle surgery is an expansive topic and these authors have done a tremendous job of anatomically breaking down the foot and ankle and giving rationale approaches to failed surgical procedures.

Failed or less than satisfactory surgical results can be disheartening to surgeons and even worse, devastating for our patients. The ability to successfully revise these complications is an art that is learned from competent mentors and colleagues, as well as from years of experience and often times heartache. Each revision case presents unique obstacles and challenges making it impossible to present everything the surgeon may encounter in this compilation or any other text. The surgeon must rely on his own acumen and prowess to plan and execute these very difficult cases properly.

Revisional surgery not only tests surgical skills but also the surgeon's ability to interact with patients. The surgeon may need to explain to a patient and their family why a previous surgery failed and why the next procedures will work. Alternatively and equally as difficult, is explaining in a professional and non provoking manner why another doctor's surgery didn't work. Good original surgery can be negated by non compliant and metabolic decrepit patients and revisional surgery in these patients must be extremely well thought out if attempted. An accurate assessment of all of the risks and benefits of revisional surgery must be weighed out, and sometimes certainly the best option is to not operate at all.

Clin Podiatr Med Surg 26 (2009) xvii–xviii
doi:10.1016/j.cpm.2008.12.002
podiatric.theclinics.com

I would like to thank the contributors for their diligence and expertise. It has been a pleasure to work with each of them. My wife and family have also been very supportive during this endeavor and I am forever grateful to them.

Jerome K. Steck, DPM, FACFAS
Southern Arizona Orthopaedics
St. Joseph's Medical Plaza II,6567 E
Carondelet Drive, Suite 415
Tucson, AZ 85710, USA

E-mail address:
jksteck@hotmail.com

Wound Complications

Monica H. Schweinberger, DPM, AACFAS, Thomas S. Roukis, DPM, PhD, FACFAS*

KEYWORDS

- Dehiscence • Postoperative infection
- Wound • Wound healing • Wound closure

In the realm of postsurgical complications, wound dehiscence may seem trivial, but can have devastating implications if not managed appropriately. Multiple factors in the preoperative, intraoperative, and postoperative period can contribute to delayed or nonhealing of surgical incisions. Therefore, surgeons must mitigate the risk factors in each of these periods to reduce the likelihood of wound healing complications. Specific attention must be paid to three distinct areas: (1) the patients' inherent risk; (2) proper surgical technique; and (3) careful postoperative management. Despite these measures, wound complications may still occur and require management with local wound care or various methods of wound closure, as discussed in this article.

HOST FACTORS

Comorbid disease processes, such as poorly controlled diabetes, peripheral arterial disease, and chronic renal failure, can significantly impact postoperative healing. Additionally, malnutrition, certain medications, and tobacco use can impair the healing process. Poorly controlled diabetes diminishes the initial inflammatory response involved in wound healing. When the inflammatory cells finally enter the surgical site, a prolonged inflammatory phase occurs that delays the deposition of matrix components, inhibits remodeling of the wound, and reduces the rate of wound closure.[1] Additionally, hyperglycemia impairs neutrophil and mononuclear phagocyte function, reducing host immune response to infection.[2] Internal medicine or endocrinology disciplines should be involved in perioperative management to aid with improved diabetic control, which should be maintained throughout healing.

Peripheral arterial disease prevents incision healing secondary to impaired oxygen delivery to the surgical site.[3] Vascular surgery should be consulted in patients who have an ankle/brachial index less than 0.7, toe pressures less than 40 mm Hg, or transcutaneous oxygen tension less than 30 mm Hg to assess the potential for endovascular or open revascularization to increase healing potential.[4]

The opinions or assertions contained herein are the private view of the author and are not to be construed as official or reflecting the views of the Department of the Army or the Department of Defense.

Limb Preservation Service, Vascular/Endovascular Surgery Service, Department of Surgery, Madigan Army Medical Center, 9040-A Fitzsimmons Avenue, MCHJ-SV, Tacoma, WA 98431, USA
* Corresponding author.
E-mail address: thomas.s.roukis@us.army.mil (T.S. Roukis).

Clin Podiatr Med Surg 26 (2009) 1–10
doi:10.1016/j.cpm.2008.09.001
0891-8422/08/$ – see front matter. Published by Elsevier Inc.

In chronic renal failure, proteinurea occurs with resultant albumin deficiency,[5] causing protein malnutrition and impaired wound healing. Additionally, patients on renal dialysis are prone to infection secondary to dysfunction of the white blood cells after contact with dialysis membranes. Resistant organisms are commonly seen in patients on dialysis because most have undergone repeated antibiotic therapy for recurrent infections at their dialysis catheter or arteriovenous fistula site. Patients on dialysis may also be exposed to contaminated fluids or waterborne bacteria during treatment, increasing the likelihood of infection.[6] Attention to detail with aseptic technique at dressing changes,[4] antibiotic prophylaxis, and nutritional supplementation is particularly important in this patient population.

Malnutrition can impair wound healing by depleting the body of metabolic energy derived from carbohydrates, proteins, and fat. Decreased intake of quality nutrition sources before surgery or injury can significantly reduce collagen synthesis.[1] Nutritional status should be assessed preoperatively through prealbumin and albumin laboratory tests. Because of its long half-life, albumin may be normal in a malnourished patient, and it is affected by a patients' hydration status, making it less accurate in assessing nutrition than prealbumin, which has a shorter half-life.[7] Patients should be encouraged to eat a well-balanced diet in addition to supplemental shakes and vitamin C for collagen synthesis. Zinc and vitamin A are recommended for patients experiencing severe stress or taking long-term steroids. Some evidence suggests that improved nutritional intake a few days before surgical intervention can increase collagen synthesis and aid in wound healing.[1]

Medications for the treatment of rheumatoid arthritis, including prednisone, methotrexate, and enbrel, have been associated with impaired wound healing or increased risk for postoperative infection. These medications are commonly tapered or discontinued perioperatively to reduce their negative effects on wound healing.

Garner and colleagues[8] evaluated the days to healing and incidence of wound complications (defined as infection, hematoma formation, and wound dehiscence) in three groups of patients undergoing orthopedic procedures: (1) rheumatoid arthritic patients receiving corticosteroids; (2) patients who had rheumatoid arthritis not receiving corticosteroids and; (3) a control group of patients who had nonrheumatoid arthritis. On average, the patients who had rheumatoid arthritis healed faster than the control group; however, the incidence of wound healing complications was greater in patients who had rheumatoid arthritis. Patients receiving corticosteroids had a significantly higher incidence of postoperative wound infection than those not receiving corticosteroids. Corticosteroids did not seem to influence hematoma formation or wound dehiscence in this study population.

A study by Jain and colleagues[9] evaluated 80 patients who had rheumatoid arthritis undergoing 129 surgical procedures of the hand and wrist over 5-years. The study compared infection and wound dehiscence rates in four groups of patients: (1) those taking prednisone alone, (2) those taking methotrexate alone, (3) those taking both drugs, and (4) those taking neither of these drugs. No statistically significant increase in wound infection or dehiscence occurred in patients taking methotrexate, prednisone, or both compared with the nonmedicated control group. However, a subgroup analysis of patients who had diabetes in addition to rheumatoid arthritis had an increased infection rate. Several studies have compared continued perioperative use of methotrexate to discontinuation of this medication before surgery, with no statistically significant difference seen in the rates of infection or wound healing complications.[9–12]

Enbrel and remicaide have been associated with postoperative wound complications because they inhibit tumor necrosis factor-α (TNF-α), which mediates the inflammatory response involved in tissue healing and infection surveillance.[13] Bibbo and colleagues[13] evaluated 31 patients who had rheumatoid arthritis undergoing elective foot and ankle surgery that were divided into two groups: (1) those being treated with TNF-α inhibitors and (2) those not receiving these medications. Equal distributions of patients in both groups were taking corticosteroids, methotrexate, leflunamide, and nonsteroidal anti-inflammatory medications perioperatively; however, group one had a six times higher proportion of smokers than group two. When considered separately, healing and infectious complications were statistically similar between the groups. Overall, the complications showed that patients in group two had a statistically significant, higher overall complication rate.[13]

Based on these data and those from other authors,[9–13] the current recommendation is to continue the use of disease-modifying antirheumatic drugs (DMARDS) and corticosteroids in the perioperative period for patients who have rheumatoid arthritis undergoing elective surgery. Nevertheless, in patients who have multiple comorbidities, such as diabetes, renal disease, or hepatic disease,[11] or those undergoing limb salvage or revision surgery, considering discontinuation or weaning of these medications in the perioperative period may be prudent despite the risk for postoperative flare. The patients' risk factors should be discussed with their rheumatologist for recommendations on weaning of steroid therapy and length of discontinuation of DMARDS, along with appropriate perioperative prophylaxis with hydrocortisone as required.

Tobacco use results in arterial spasm, which can impair oxygen delivery to healing tissues. Additionally, chemicals from inhaled cigarette smoke break down vitamin C, which can reduce collagen synthesis and delay wound healing.[14] Patients scheduled to undergo elective surgery should be encouraged to discontinue smoking and be referred to a smoking cessation program. Surgeons prefer that patients abstain from tobacco use before surgery, but the duration of preoperative abstinence required to reduce wound healing complications has not been definitively determined. Use of nicotine transdermal patches has not been extensively studied with regard to wound healing complications, although studies that have been performed have not shown increased risk for wound healing complications in these patients compared with nontobacco users.

Fulcher and colleagues[15] evaluated microvascular responses to cold temperatures in 10 chronic tobacco users before cessation and at 2 and 7 days after tobacco cessation and compared them with nontobacco user controls. Within 7 days after tobacco cessation, digital microvascular perfusion normalized in the subjects who used nicotine transdermal patches and those who did not,[15] suggesting either that nicotine is not responsible for changes in microvascular function or that the amount of nicotine in the patch is not sufficient to affect the microcirculation.[16]

Sorensen and colleagues[17] evaluated collagen synthesis on polytetrafluoroethylene tubing implanted into the subcutaneous tissue in 54 tobacco users who abstained from tobacco use for 20 days. After 10 days, half of the tobacco users were randomized to receive a 25 mg/d transdermal nicotine patch and the control group was administered a placebo transdermal patch. The nicotine transdermal patch group had an 18% increase in type I procollagen on explanted tubing, whereas the placebo group had a 10% decrease, indicating that the nicotine transdermal patch may increase type I collagen synthesis.[17] Nicotine transdermal patches help people abstain from tobacco use longer, and are probably helpful during recovery after surgery to prevent relapse.[16]

SURGICAL TECHNIQUE

Many technical factors during surgery can significantly impact postoperative wound healing. Implementing protocols that can reduce the risk for postoperative infection are of primary importance. In 1980, Cruse and Foord[18] published a prospective epidemiologic study evaluating postoperative infection rates at a teaching hospital over 10 years. Multiple risk factors for postoperative infection were identified and remedied, reducing the hospital's postoperative infection rates.

Several recommendations resulted from the findings of this study that are still valid today. To reduce the bacterial load on the patients' skin, a preoperative shower with hexachlorophene was performed that decreased infection rates from 13% to 2.3% in clean wounds. Patients who were hospitalized for extended periods before surgery were noted to have increased postoperative infection rates probably from bacterial colonization on their skin. Although the authors recommended a shorter hospital stay,[18] this is not possible in some instances.

Currently, this article's senior author's (TSR) inpatient protocol includes a daily whole-body Hibiclens (Chlorhexidine Gluconate Solution, 4%, Cardinal Health, McGaw Park, IL) sponge bath which results in a sustained antibacterial effect with multiple uses,[19] reducing bacterial colonization.

Shaving before surgery has been shown to increase infection rates secondary to skin excoriations in which bacterial colonization occurs.[20] Therefore, any shaving (or preferably use of a depilatory) is recommended to be performed in the operating room immediately before the procedure to reduce the time available for bacteria to invade the area.[18]

Careful surgical preparation of the skin is especially important for avoiding postoperative infection. Keblish and colleagues[21] showed that use of a scrub brush in addition to an isopropyl alcohol paint significantly reduced the number of colony-forming units of bacteria on the skin after surgical preparation of the foot and ankle. The combination of a 4% chlorhexidine gluconate scrub followed by a 70% isopropyl alcohol paint has been shown to be most effective at eliminating bacterial contamination of the skin.[19]

Prophylactic antibiotics have been associated with a reduction in the rate of postoperative infection.[22] Studies have shown some usefulness even in clean surgeries for immunocompromised patients if a prosthesis is inserted, or when extensive soft-tissue dissection is required that may result in diminished blood supply to the surgical site.[2,22] In revision surgery, antibiotic prophylaxis would be recommended because of increased operative time and greater likelihood of devascularization at the surgical site with a second procedure. The type of antibiotic used should be safe, have a narrow spectrum of coverage for the most likely pathogen, not be used in the clinical treatment of infection to prevent development of resistance, and be administered either for one dose or a maximum of 24 hours. Because most surgical site infections in clean surgery are caused by *Staphylococcus aureus* and *S epidermidis*, a first-generation cephalosporin is preferred, with clindamycin or vancomycin used in patients who have a penicillin allergy.[2]

Several studies have correlated a rise in infection rates with increasing operative time,[18,23,24] with four likely reasons: (1) bacterial contamination is more likely to occur the longer a surgical site remains open; (2) desiccation of the wound and excessive retraction with prolonged operative time can damage cellular components at the incision site; (3) excessive use of electrocautery or suture material leaves residual necrotic tissue and foreign material within the incision site, increasing the likelihood of infection; and (4) patients may have decreased resistance to infection secondary to increased blood loss and the potential for shock with prolonged procedures.[18] Expeditious use of surgical time, termed *economy of motion*, is therefore necessary to reduce the likelihood of postoperative wound complications. Surgeons must prepare for the procedure and ensure that all instrumentation, dressings, and other surgical equipment are readily accessible or open on the field before beginning surgery to reduce the number of delays during the case and thereby decrease operative time.

When performing any surgical procedure, incision placement parallel to the relaxed skin tension lines is preferred[25] to allow good apposition of the incision without tension on wound closure. Meticulous dissection with use of full-thickness skin flaps when possible helps to preserve the vascular supply and reduce the likelihood of wound dehiscence or necrosis at the incision line.[26] When exposing bone to perform an osteotomy or apply fixation, using a periosteal elevator to lift the periosteum along with the overlying soft-tissue as a unit reduces trauma to the cutaneous vascular supply and results in fewer wound complications postoperatively. The skin should be carefully retracted to avoid crushing the tissue. An example would be using a forceps with multiple teeth (ie, Adson Brown forceps) rather than one with two or three teeth, because a forceps with multiple teeth allows easy manipulation of the tissue without the need to firmly clamp down on it, thereby minimizing trauma. Meticulous hemostasis must be achieved with the use of vascular clips (Ligaclip 20/20 multiple clip applier, Ethicon Endo-surgery, Inc., Cincinnati, Ohio), electrocautery, or suture material, which should all be used sparingly if possible. Blood is an excellent medium for bacterial growth, and therefore hematoma formation must be avoided. A drain should be placed if sustained drainage is expected, but should always exit the surgical site through a separate stab incision, rather than the surgical incision itself to reduce the risk of contiguous spread of infection.[18] The drain should be maintained until output is less than 1cc per hour over a 24 hour period after which it can be removed.

Wound closure should be performed without tension and with slight eversion of the skin edges to achieve gentle re-approximation of the incision.[27] Sutures should be placed starting at the midline of the incision and then at half way points between the initial suture and the end point of the incision to avoid standing cutaneous defects (ie, dog ears). This is followed by intermittent metallic skin staples between the sutures to achieve complete wound closure. If the skin edges become blanched after wound closure, sutures and/or staples should be sequentially removed until normal capillary refill returns. Following this, wound closure can be achieved through: (1) use of fewer, more widely spaced sutures; (2) creation of a V-Y fasciocutaneous flap to advance adjacent tissue and achieve tension free closure; (3) coverage using a split- or full-thickness skin graft harvested from regional tissues; or (4) the wound can be left open to granulate in with or without application of negative pressure therapy. The senior author (TSR) routinely uses widely spaced vertical mattress sutures of 2-0 nylon interposed by staples for skin closure. The vertical mattress suture provides eversion of the skin edges which promotes primary healing. The nylon suture is minimally reactive and the large size needle is easy to manipulate and allows controlled passage through the tissues without traumatizing them. Metallic skin staples are minimally reactive, are used in addition to sutures to allow complete approximation of the incision and are the first to be removed during the postoperative period. The ability to alternate between removal of the metallic skin staples and sutures allows gradually increasing stress to be placed on the wound edges over time which affords durable maturation and minimizes dehiscence.

POSTOPERATIVE MANAGEMENT

Incision healing is dependent upon a few key factors in the postoperative period: (1) edema control; (2) immobilization; and (3) a clean environment. Continuous limb elevation above heart level with a maximum of 30 minutes of dependency at a time for meals and icing behind the knee 15 minutes per hour while the patient is awake can limit the development of edema and reduce tension on the skin edges. The senior author (TSR) uses a modified Jones compression dressing postoperatively to aid with edema control and immobilization of the extremity. Use of a sugar tong splint or cast over the dressing provides additional immobilization which can be especially helpful with healing of incisions about the ankle that are subject to significant stress with ankle movement. Posterior splints are avoided to reduce the risk of developing posterior heel and forefoot ulcers which can be devastating, especially in high-risk patients.

Patients with significant risk for wound dehiscence should be kept non-weight bearing until complete incision healing has occurred, even if they have only undergone a soft-tissue procedure. If weightbearing is allowed, it should be significantly limited (ie, 25 steps per day) and rolling off the forefoot should be prevented. Dressing changes should exclusively be performed by the physician's involved in the patients care at postoperative visits and the patients' foot and leg should be cleansed with an antibacterial solution (Technicare surgical scrub, Care-Tech Laboratories, Inc., Saint Louis, MO) at each change to reduce the bacterial load on the skin and subsequently lower the risk of postoperative infection.[4] Institution of this dressing protocol by the senior author (TSR) has been effective at reducing infection rates in patients with chronic foot and ankle wounds[19] and in preventing pin tract infections in patients treated with external fixation.[28] Patients must perform daily sponge baths to keep the dressing dry and avoid condensation underneath which can cause maceration and skin breakdown.

Sutures and/or staples should be left in place until the incision is fully healed as long as they are continuing to provide support at the surgical site. This can require 4 weeks or longer in some cases. A portion of the staples and sutures can be taken out over a series of visits, to allow the incision line to mature before complete removal, as described above.

WOUND DEHISCENCE

Delayed and non-healing of incisions can occur despite careful pre-, intra-, and post-operative management of the patient. In treating this complication it is important to reassess the patient and carefully evaluate the wound to determine the reasons for wound dehiscence and address them, in addition to considering options for wound healing or wound closure. The patients' vascular status should be re-evaluated to ensure that their pulses remain palpable, or that any previous endovascular intervention or bypass procedure continues to supply adequate blood flow to the surgical site. Any change in vascular status should prompt referral to a vascular surgeon. Hyperbaric oxygen may be considered for patients who are not candidates for revascularization.[29]

Infection resulting in wound dehiscence should be managed with oral or intravenous antibiosis. In severe infections, an irrigation and debridement may be required with removal of all necrotic tissue using a scalpel, curette and/or a hydrosurgery tool (Versejet, Smith and Nephew, Key Largo, FL) for more precise debridement.[30] Pulse lavage irrigation should be performed with 3 L of normal saline plain, followed by gram stain, aerobic and anaerobic cultures, to determine if any bacteria are left in the wound, and then 3 L of normal saline mixed with one or more antibiotics. Polymethylmethacrylate antibiotic loaded cement beads can be placed for sterilization of the wound and are generally removed in 48–72 hours. If there are still signs of infection or necrotic tissue is present, repeat debridement with antibiotic bead exchange should be performed until the wound is completely clean.

Once the infection has been cleared the residual wound must be assessed to determine if closure by secondary intent is indicated or if other viable options for wound closure could be attempted. The "reconstructive elevator" provides a list of these options including: (1) delayed primary closure with or without continuous tension devices or tissue expansion; (2) split- or full-thickness skin grafting; (3) adjacent tissue re-arrangement or random-pattern local flaps; (4) distant (ie, pedicled) composite flaps; and (5) free tissue transfer with microvascular anastomosis.[31,32]

Superficial wounds can be closed by secondary intent using debridement every 10–14 days with careful attention to remove any peri-wound hyperkeratotic tissue which can splint the wound open. Enzymatic débridement agents such as Panafil ointment (Healthpoint, Ltd., Fort Worth, TX) or Accuzyme ointment (Healthpoint Ltd., Fort Worth, TX) may be used if sharp débridement has not adequately removed fibrous or necrotic tissue from the wound bed.[33] Once granular tissue is present, the wound should be kept moist with application of hydrogels such as Silvasorb gel (Medline Industries, Inc., Mundelein, IL). Collagen matrices like Promogran Matrix Wound Dressing (Johnson & Johnson Medical Limited, Gargrave, Skipton, U.K.), Prisma Matrix Wound Dressing (Johnson & Johnson Medical Limited, Gargrave, Skipton, U.K.), or gel foam may be used in conjunction with a hydrogel or platelet derived growth factor (Regranex Gel 0.01%, Ethicon, Inc., Somerville, NJ) to stimulate more rapid healing.[34] Steri-strips may aid in reducing tension across the wound and help with re-approximation of the skin edges.

Biological dressings such as Graftjacket Ulcer Repair Matrix (Wright Medical Technology, Inc., Arlington TN) and Unite Biomatrix (Pegasus Biologics, Inc., Irvine, CA) can be applied over clean granular wounds and secured with skin staples. An antibiotic ointment and non-adherent petroleum based dressing are then applied over these tissues to maintain hydration. The biological dressing is left in place until it either becomes incorporated into the wound or desiccates at which point it is removed, usually at about 4 weeks after application. The underlying wound will generally be significantly smaller, or in some cases, fully healed at this point. Any remaining open wound is usually treated with local wound care measures as described above until complete healing.

Smaller wound dehiscence's can be treated with delayed primary closure under sterile technique after freshening the skin edges. For larger wounds, continuous tension devices (ie, skin expanders) such as the ABRA Dynamic Wound Closure system (Canica Design, Inc., Almonte, Ontario Canada) can be used to gradually pull the wound edges together by exploiting the normal viscoelastic properties of skin (ie, mechanical creep).[35] These devices provide continuous tension on the wound edges and are sequentially tightened over time to gradually re-approximate the wounds edges until they can be primarily closed.

Deep or tunneling wounds can benefit from the use of negative pressure therapy (Wound V.A.C. Therapy Systems, San Antonio, TX) to stimulate granulation tissue formation, reduce bacterial load and cause wound contracture. Living cell therapy such as Apligraf (Organogenesis, Inc., Canton, MA)[36] or topical growth factors such as Regranex Gel 0.01% (Ethicon, Inc., Somerville, NJ) can be used in isolation or in combination with negative pressure therapy to speed formation of healthy granulation tissue. Once a healthy granular bed is present and flush with the surrounding skin edges, a split-thickness skin graft can be applied. The senior author (TSR) uses platelet rich plasma in combination with split-thickness skin grafting which allows immediate fibrin anchorage of the graft to the wound bed followed by either a simple staple-over bolster dressing composed of non-adherent petroleum gauze and saline soaked cotton balls stapled in place over the graft[37] or negative pressure therapy over the site until good take is appreciated.[38] The patient is admitted and placed on bed rest until the skin graft is assessed at 5 days postoperative. If the graft is well adhered, the bolster dressing is usually discontinued and replaced with antibiotic ointment and non-adherent petroleum based gauze along with re-application of a Jones compression dressing and sugar tong splint. If the skin graft fails, local wound care is reinstituted to allow closure by secondary intent or to prepare the wound for another attempt at coverage.

If metallic hardware is exposed in the wound but providing stable osseous fixation, early coverage with a local advancement flap, pedicled flap, or intrinsic foot muscle flap[39] in conjunction with split-thickness skin grafting may be considered dependent on the location and size of the wound, as well as, the vascular status of the patient. Patients with peripheral arterial disease, even after revascularization, are generally poor candidates for flap coverage due to the likely presence of microvascular disease. Loose or unstable metallic hardware should be removed and replaced with an external fixator, if required, for osseous support. Free tissue transfer with microvascular anastomosis can be considered for deep or more extensive wounds, which would require a reconstructive plastic surgery consult.[40] If flaps are performed, the patient must be hospitalized on bed rest to allow regular monitoring for arterial inflow and venous congestion until the flap is stable, usually 5–7 days or longer. Careful attention must be paid to avoid compression of the flap which can lead to necrosis. Use of an external fixator as a "kickstand" to off-load the posterior heel has been described and may be useful for flaps to this area.[41] External fixation can also be used for immobilization of the limb and allow for easier access to the wound for dressing changes or monitoring of a flap, without the need to repeatedly remove and re-apply splints.[42]

SUMMARY

Wound complications are difficult to manage and can significantly prolong a patients recovery from surgery. When infection is present or significant tissue loss with metallic hardware exposure occurs, these complications can become limb threatening. Measures taken in the perioperative period can help to reduce the incidence of wound dehiscence but do not completely eliminate the problem. A systematic approach to the treatment of these wounds must be used with the primary goal of eradicating any infection present. Once this has been accomplished the patient and their wound must be carefully evaluated to determine etiologic factors that can be remedied to aid healing. Ultimately, multiple options for wound closure can be undertaken ranging from healing by secondary intent through flap coverage dependent on the size, location, and type of wound.

REFERENCES

1. Arnold M, Barbul A. Nutrition and wound healing. Plast Reconstr Surg 2006; 117(7S):42S–58S.
2. Barie PS, Eachempati SR. Surgical site infections. Surg Clin North Am 2005;85: 1115–35.
3. Hagino RT. Vascular assessment and reconstruction of the ischemic diabetic limb. Clin Podiatr Med Surg 2007;24(3):449–67.
4. Andersen CA, Roukis TS. The diabetic foot. Surg Clin North Am 2007;87(5): 1149–77.
5. Murdoch DP, Armstrong DG, Cacus JB, et al. The natural history of great toe amputations. J Foot Ankle Surg 1997;36(3):204–6.
6. Berman SJ. Infections in patients with end-stage renal disease. An overview. Infect Dis Clin North Am 2001;15(3):709–20.
7. Gomella LG, Haist SA, Billeter M. Diets and clinical nutrition. In: Gomella LG, Haist SA, Billeter M, editors. Clinicians pocket reference. 8th edition. Stamford (CT): Appleton & Lange; 1997. p. 189.

8. Garner RW, Mowat AG, Hazleman BL. Wound healing after operations on patients with rheumatoid arthritis. J Bone Joint Surg Br 1973;55(1):134–44.
9. Jain A, Witbreuk M, Ball C, et al. Influence of steroids and methotrexate on wound complications after elective rheumatoid hand and wrist surgery. J Hand Surg [Am] 2002;27(3):449–55.
10. Murata K, Yasuda T, Ito H, et al. Lack of increase in postoperative complications with low-dose methotrexate therapy in patients with rheumatoid arthritis undergoing elective orthopedic surgery. Mod Rheumatol 2006;16(1):14–9.
11. Pieringer H, Stuby U, Biesenbach G. Patients with rheumatoid arthritis undergoing surgery: how should we deal with antirheumatic treatment? Semin Arthritis Rheum 2007;36(5):278–86.
12. Kasdan ML, June L. Postoperative results of rheumatoid arthritis patients on methotrexate at the time of reconstructive surgery of the hand. Orthopedics 1993;16(11):1233–5.
13. Bibbo C, Goldberg JW. Infectious and healing complications after elective orthopaedic foot and ankle surgery during tumor necrosis factor-alpha inhibition therapy. Foot Ankle Int 2004;25(5):331–5.
14. Hemalatha A, Venkatesan A, Bobby Z, et al. Antioxidant response to oxidative stress induced by smoking. Indian J Physiol Pharmacol 2006;50(4):416–20.
15. Fulcher SM, Koman LA, Smith BP, et al. The effect of transdermal nicotine on digital perfusion in reformed habitual smokers. J Hand Surg [Am] 1998;23(5):792–9.
16. Warner DO. Perioperative abstinence from cigarettes. Physiologic and clinical consequences. Anesthesiology 2006;104(2):356–67.
17. Sorensen LT, Jorgensen LN, Zillmer R, et al. Transdermal nicotine patch enhances type I collagen synthesis in abstinent smokers. Wound Repair Regen 2006;14(3):247–51.
18. Cruse PJE, Foord R. The epidemiology of wound infection. A 10-year prospective study of 62,939 wounds. Surg Clin North Am 1980;60(1):27–40.
19. Schade VL, Roukis TS. Use of a surgical prep and sterile dressing during office visit treatment of chronic foot and ankle wounds decreases the incidence of infection and treatment costs. The Foot and Ankle Specialist 2008;1(3):147–54.
20. Seropian R, Reynolds BM. Wound infections after preoperative depilatory versus razor preparation. Am J Surg 1971;121(3):251–4.
21. Keblish DJ, Zurakowski D, Wilson MG, et al. Preoperative skin preparation of the foot and ankle: bristles and alcohol are better. J Bone Joint Surg Am 2005;87(5):986–92.
22. Sandusky WR. Use of prophylactic antibiotics in surgical patients. Surg Clin North Am 1980;60(1):83–92.
23. Cohen LS, Fekety FR Jr, Cluff LE. Studies of the epidemiology of staphylococcal infection: VI. Infections in the surgical patient. Ann Surg 1964;159(3):321–34.
24. Williams RE, McDonald JC, Blowers R, The Public Health Laboratory Service. Incidence of surgical wound infection in England and Wales: a report of the public health laboratory service. Lancet 1960;2:659–63.
25. Mahan KT. Plastic surgery and skin grafting. In: McGlamry ED, Banks AS, Downey MS, editors. 2nd edition. Comprehensive textbook of foot surgery. vol. 2. Philadelphia: Williams & Wilkins; 1992. p. 1256–8.
26. Pyka RA, Coventry MB. Avascular necrosis of the skin after operations on the foot. J Bone Joint Surg Am 1961;43(7):955–60.
27. Multhopp-Stephens H, Michael RH. A skin suture for foot and ankle surgery. Foot Ankle Int 1994;15(7):404–5.

28. Schweinberger M, Roukis TS. The effectiveness of physician directed external fixation pin site care in preventing pin site infection in a high-risk patient population. In: Programs and abstracts of the American College of Foot and Ankle Surgeons Annual Scientific Conference. Long Beach, 21 February 2008. p. 60.
29. Niinikoski JHA. Clinical hyperbaric oxygen therapy, wound perfusion, and transcutaneous oximetry. World J Surg 2004;28(3):307–11.
30. Klein MB, Hunter S, Heimbach DM, et al. The Versajet™ water dissector: a new tool for tangential excision. J Burn Care Rehabil 2005;26(6):483–7.
31. Levin LS. The reconstructive ladder: an ortho-plastic approach. Orthop Clin North Am 1993;24(3):393–409.
32. Bennett N, Choudhary S. Why climb a ladder when you can take the elevator? Plast Reconstr Surg 2000;105(6):2266.
33. Ramundo J, Gray M. Enzymatic wound debridement. J Wound Ostomy Continence Nurs 2008;35(3):273–80.
34. Fonder MA, Lazarus GS, Cowan DA, et al. Treating the chronic wound: a practical approach to the care of non-healing wounds and wound care dressings. J Am Acad Dermatol 2008;58(2):185–206.
35. Concannon MJ, Puckett CL. Wound coverage using modified tissue expansion. Plast Reconstr Surg 1998;102(2):377–84.
36. Karr J. Utilization of living bilayered cell therapy (Apligraf) for heel ulcers. Adv Skin Wound Care 2008;21(6):270–4.
37. Roukis TS. Radical solutions. Bold debridement techniques can work for both chronic and acute wounds. OrthoKinetic Rev 2004;4(1):20–3.
38. Stone P, Prigozen J, Hofeldt M, et al. Bolster versus negative pressure wound therapy for securing split-thickness skin grafts in trauma patients. Wounds 2004;16(7):219–23.
39. Levin LS. Foot and ankle soft-tissue deficiencies: who needs a flap? Am J Orthop 2006;35(1):11–9.
40. Hallock GG, Arangio GA. Free-flap salvage of soft tissue complications following the lateral approach to the calcaneus. Ann Plast Surg 2007;58(2):179–81.
41. Roukis TS, Landsman AS, Weinberg SA, et al. Use of a hybrid "kickstand" external fixator for pressure relief after soft-tissue reconstruction of heel defects. J Foot Ankle Surg 2003;42(4):240–3.
42. Oznur A, Zgonis T. Closure of major diabetic foot wounds and defects with external fixation. Clin Podiatr Med Surg 2007;24(3):519–28.

Revisional Peripheral Nerve Surgery

Jarrett D. Cain, DPM, MSc, AACFAS[a], Kris DiNucci, DPM, FACFAS[b,*]

KEYWORDS

- Neuroma • Compressive neuropathies • Revision surgery
- Neurolysis • Nerve wrapping • Nerve grafts • Nerve adjuncts

There are variety of peripheral nerve disorders that exist in the foot and ankle. Some of the common conditions can be categorized as neuroma, compressive neuropathies, and diabetic neuropathy.

NEUROMA

Originally described in 1845,[1] neuroma describes a painful condition of the common plantar nerves of the interspace of the forefoot. Although the term "neuroma" is popularly used to define the condition, other terms, such as "neuralgia," "neurtitis," "perineural fibrosis," and "interdigital neuritis" have been used to describe the condition as well.[1–5] Neuromas secondary to trauma have also been reported.[6]

Compressive Neuropathies

Patients with compressive neuropathies commonly present with diffuse pain secondary to nerve compression or entrapment within a tunnel or fibro-osseous space.[7] One of the more common entrapment/compressive neuropathies is tarsal tunnel syndrome (TTS), which is compression of the tibial nerve within the tarsal canal behind the medial malleolus.[8] Other compressive neuropathies have been reported within the foot and ankle, such as the deep peroneal nerve[9] as it travels with the dorsalis pedis artery beneath the inferior extensor retinaculum in the anterior aspect of the ankle and at the dorsal midfoot. Sural and saphenous nerves have been reported to be compressed along their course as well.[10]

In patients with long-standing heel pain, entrapment of the first branch of the lateral plantar nerve, also called "Baxter's nerve," may occur as it travels between the abductor hallucis muscle and quadratus plantae muscle.[11,12]

[a] 1444 New Haven, Cary, Illinois 60013, USA
[b] Foot and Ankle Center of Arizona, 7312 E. Deer Valley Road, Suite 110, Scottsdale, AZ 85255-7452, USA
* Corresponding author.
E-mail address: k4din@aol.com (K. DiNucci).

Clin Podiatr Med Surg 26 (2009) 11–22
doi:10.1016/j.cpm.2008.10.002
podiatric.theclinics.com
0891-8422/08/$ – see front matter

Diabetic Neuropathy

Introduced by Dellon,[13] the theory of diabetic neuropathy is based on external nerve compression interrupting axonal blood flow. Release of the peripheral nerve compression sites is believed to restore axonal blood flow, relieve pain, and restore sensation. Although it has shown clinical promise based on previous studies, this procedure has not been widely accepted as a standard treatment for diabetic neuropathy.

Nerve disorders can cause pathologic problems, such as loss of sensation, loss of motor function, pain, autonomic changes, and other various symptoms. A variety of operative techniques are employed to relieve patients' symptoms. However, when these techniques fail to provide relief, chronic pain can persist, creating hindrances in the daily lifestyle of the patient. Reports have shown it is not uncommon for poor outcomes to arise with peripheral nerve surgery and create chronic symptoms for the patient. The clinician must identify factors associated with direct causes of chronic nerve pain. These factors can be categorized as internal or external factors.[14] Internal factors (ie, nerve damage secondary to injury or trauma, myelin degeneration, axon damage) are related to changes within the nerve tissue that contribute to patients symptoms, while external factors are the outside contributions (ie, biomechanical factors, space occupying lesion, narrow fibro-osseus tunnel), which create chronic nerve disorders. Internal factors that affect peripheral nerves create symptoms that either include spontaneous discharges of the nerve that eliciting severe pain, known as ectopic neuralgia, or can generate severe pain on palpation or activity, known as nociceptive neuralgia.[15]

In evaluating external factors, nerve compression anywhere along the course of the peripheral nerves may cause symptoms in the lower extremities. These sites include the common peroneal nerve at the fibular neck, the posterior tibial nerve at the medial ankle and the posterior tibial nerve bifurcation site at the abductor hiatus, the deep peroneal nerve at the dorsal midfoot, and the superficial peroneal nerve at the anterolateral leg. A positive clinical finding of nerve irriation or compression is noted by the presence of a Tinel's sign on percussion of the nerve at the compression site. A positive Tinel's sign is consistent with nerve pathology and may reveal current disease to the nerve, a narrow fibro-osseus tunnel, or a systemic disease state contributing to the nerve condition. The sensation of the peripheral nerve course along with the lumbar and sacral dermatomal distribution should be analyzed. A loss or decrease in sensation in the anatomic region of a peripheral nerve root should lead to the suspicion of lumbar nerve root pathology. It is important that they not only be recognized but a distinction be made between the two types of factors.

An often-overlooked common external factor is double crush syndrome. Double crush syndrome occurs when a patient has a proximal nerve compression that alters axonal transport and may contribute to a secondary distal entrapment. Double crush syndrome was originally described by Upton and McComas,[16] who observed that 70% of their patients who had symptomatic carpal tunnel and ulnar neuropathy had evidence of cervical root lesions. They believed that there was an increased association of symptomatic patients and those with proximal constraints and metabolic abnormalities, such as diabetes.[16] As a result, the patient experiences decreased axoplasmic flow, which predisposes the nerve to dysfunction.[17] These compressions are thought to compromise nerve function by altering the axonal transport delivery system, which is critical to nerve function. If unrecognized, patients undergoing surgical release of a peripheral nerve entrapment may only have mild or transient relief of the presenting symptoms.

REVISIONAL SURGICAL PATIENT EVALUATION

When evaluating a patient for chronic neurologic pain, a comprehensive evaluation must be undertaken to provide insight as to why the primary surgical correction was unsuccessful. Factors to be considered include identification of the specific nerve involved and review of prior nonoperative and operative intervention. Important questions that must be answered during the evaluation are:

- Are there any systemic diseases associated with the patient's condition?
- Does the patient have an underlying biomechanical factor associated with the chronic pain?
- Did the patient have any contributions from previous trauma to the area that may contribute to the symptoms?
- Was the initial diagnosis of the patient's symptoms correct?
- Is there a difference between the initial and current symptoms experienced by the patient?
- Did the patient experience any resolution of initial symptoms, whether it was full, partial, or not at all?

A thorough evaluation, including physical examination, imaging, laboratory, and electrico-diagnostic studies is necessary to assure the proper diagnosis before intervention. It is common for the surgeon to obtain a limited evaluation and testing of the patient before performing repeat surgery. The characteristics involving the nerve pain must be identified through a complete foot, ankle, and lower extremity examination. Patients with chronic peripheral neuropathy symptoms will commonly present with complaints of intermittent burning-type pain, numbness, and paresthesias, which is initially generalized and vague. This symptomatology may be localized to the distribution of the peripheral nerve or multiple nerves. Pain from a compression neuropathy is commonly accentuated by activity and worsens at the end of the day. As the compression progresses, night pain may manifest and is thought to represent nocturnal ischemia.

In the neurologic examination, testing should begin with the origin of the peripheral nerves at the lumbar spine. The location of the nerve symptoms may not be related to local nerve pathology within the foot or ankle. Pathology of the lower back with lumbar nerve root compression because of a herniated disc may be the primary etiology of symptoms in the feet or toes, regardless of the presences of symptoms in the lower back. Lumbar nerve root compression in the lumbar spine can be assessed with either a straight leg-raise test or a slump test. The slump test is a reliable indicator in the diagnosis of lumbar nerve root impingement.[18] The slump test is a modification of the straight leg-raise test and is performed in the seated position. It is a progressive series of maneuvers designed to place the sciatic nerve roots under increasing tension. Patients with a positive test will require further evaluation by a physician trained in the treatment of spinal disorders.

Clincal examination may reveal hypoesthesia to pin-prick and light touch may be appreciated. Percussion of the peripheral nerve at a site of compression may elicit paresthesias in the distribution of the injured nerve (Tinel's sign). Occasionally, in more advanced cases, nerve trunk tenderness to direct pressure with proximal and distal radiation of symptoms (Valleix's Sign) may be elicited. In the diagnosis of TTS, the use of a venous tourniquet may assist in the diagnosis of venous congestion as an etiologic factor in the pathogenesis.[19] Other investigators have proposed biomechanical mechanisms to the symptoms of TTS, with the recreation of pain with inversion and eversion of the foot.[20] As the compression of the tarsal tunnel continues, motor weakness of the intrinsics may occur. Loss of the intrinsics may be tested by having the patient fan their toes apart or by the presentation of multiple contraction of the digits.

There are many biomechanical and joint conditions of the lower extremity that may aggravate adjacent nerves, so it is imperative to perform a thorough biomechanical assessment to include range-of-motion, manual muscle testing, palpation of joints, and a static weight-bearing and gait examination. Abnormalities of the biomechanical examination should be addressed with the use of orthotics, braces, or supportive shoes as necessary. Tests that can be performed include radiologic studies, electrodiagnostic studies, and peripheral nerve blocks. Radiologic studies are helpful to diagnose biomechanical effects on nerve pathology, along with any bone abnormalities, fractures, or external space-occupying lesions. Weight-bearing foot and ankle radiographs are helpful to evaluate the presence of joint arthrosis, biomechanical abnormalities, or bone prominences as a primary source of the patient's symptoms or by contributing to peripheral nerve compression.

Electrodiagnostic studies can be helpful in determining the quality of the nerve being examined, along with determining the presence of active pathology to the nerve. Nerve conduction studies (motor, sensory, or mixed) evaluate the function of a particular nerve by electrically stimulating the nerve.[21] The clinical response is compared with normative data, based on the specific nerve at a specific site. This test can yield useful information about axonal loss and demyelination.[21] The nerve conduction velocity is determined by dividing the distance by the conduction time (latency). External neural pressure initially results in focal demyelination. The degree of nerve conduction velocity slowing and the presence of secondary axonal changes are helpful in grading the severity of the nerve compression.[21] These studies have been reported to have questionable impact on the type of revisional procedure that is performed.[22]

It is important for the clinician to read studies in light of the full examination and not rely solely on the results from electrodiagnostic studies, because of incidence of false-negatives. Budek and colleagues[23] performed nerve conduction studies on 28 patients with pes planus. The results demonstrated mild-prolongation distal latency of the medial- and lateral-plantar sensory nerves, and delayed sensory conduction velocity of the medial-plantar sensory nerve. The presence of electrodiagnostic abnormalities in this study population helps to substantiate the presence of compression neuropathy of the medial- or lateral-plantar nerve in pes planus subjects. Bailie and Keilikan, over a 10-year period, examined 47 patients who underwent surgical management for TTS.[24] All patients had nonsurgical care for an average of 16 months before surgery. The symptom triad of pain, paresthesias, and numbness was the most common clinical presentation. All had a positive Tinel's sign and nerve compression test at the tarsal tunnel; however, electrodiagnostic studies were abnormal in only 38 feet (81%).

A nerve block provides insight on the degree of nerve damage, which may be present in the patient by isolating the nerve. The use of a local anesthetic (lidocaine or bupivicaine) diagnostic block can help determine whether revision transection of the nerve or specific nerve branches could be successful in eliminating pain.[25] An additional test that has been reported to provide a sensory test of peripheral nerve function is a Pressure Sensory Specific Device (PSSD).[26] Although there have been limited studies reported, the PSSD is designed to measure one-point and two-point sensory pressure thresholds and two-point minimum space thresholds.

REVISION SURGERY TREATMENTS

The primary reason for revisional surgery is inadequate nerve release in the primary procedure. Careful attention must be directed at the incision site of the original procedure, as well as obtaining pertinent clinical and surgical reports of the patient's care. The surgical description is very important to determine if adequate exposure or decompression was performed during the primary surgical procedure.[22] This could also be important to determine if there is any hyperpathia or dysthesia present along the incision and along the course of the nerve.

Assuming the correct diagnosis was made, the next predictor of a successful outcome is the correct performance of the surgical procedure. If the procedure fails to completely address the external compression, creating the neuropathic symptoms in entrapment neuropathies or adequately resect stump neuromas, these procedures may provide either partial or no relief. Proper surgical technique addresses superficial and deep fascial structures, narrow fibroosseus tunnels, and tendon coursing over the nerves. These are important structures which require complete release.

Pathologic changes induced by nerve adhesions must also be considered in revisional situations. Degenerative changes or scarring of the nerve bed may occur because of trauma, surgery, repetitive motion, or systemic diseases, such as diabetes or rheumatoid arthritis.[27] These changes disrupt the gliding moment of the nerve and create neuro-fibrosis. Reduction of the intraneural blood flow from such scarring surrounding intraneural vessels causes ischemic changes in interfascicular tissue. The nerves become less elastic and more vulnerable to pressure.

When treating peripheral nerve pathology, consideration must be given to the unique anatomy of nerve movement. Loss on the gliding function is critical to provide the most optimal outcome in revisional nerve surgery. In peripheral nerve surgery, the formation of scar tissue is detrimental and if the nerve is inadequately released, it will limit the extent of the patient's recovery and pain relief. The nerve's gliding function is paramount to preventing adhesions to the surrounding tissue postoperatively. The paraneurium, as described by Millesi,[28] contains special gliding tissue, which allows easy dissection and mobilization of a nerve. When the gliding apparatus is lost the nerve becomes adherent to its surroundings.

The environment of a bloodless field and the use of magnification, bipolar coagulation, and intraoperative electrical stimulation of the nerve provide optimal intraoperative conditions during revisional nerve surgery.[29] When evaluating the quality of the nerve intraoperatively, Fontana's bands can help to determine the health of the peripheral nerve. In 1779, Felice Fontana described what appeared to be spiral bands surrounding peripheral nerves. These bands have been considered as representing nerve fiber undulation and can be seen readily through the epineurium as healthy nerve. Dellon observed that Fontana's bands could not be seen when the median nerve was inspected during carpal tunnel decompression, while the bands often returned following intraneural neurolysis.[30] Research performed by Abe colleagues[31] in experimental peripheral nerve adhesion in rabbits confirms that the disappearance of Fontana's bands appears to be a fairly reliable indicator of nerve fibrosis. Numerous causes have been described creating fibrosis of peripheral nerves following surgery, such as external compression, edema, hematoma, and ischemia.[32]

Neurolysis

Common surgical options for treatment of compression neuropathies in the foot and ankle include decompression or external neurolysis at the site of entrapment and, infrequently, internal neurolysis. When performing neurolysis on a nerve densely adherent to surrounding structures, one must ensure that longitudinal excursion will be restored postoperatively. If the local environment remains unaltered, adhesions will recur and clinical symptoms are likely to persist or return. The success rates of primary neurolysis surgery in compressive neuropathies has been well documented. However, when primary neurolysis does not yield success, there are circumstances when revision nerve surgery in the form of a secondary neurolysis needs to be performed. The results from surgical correction from this condition vary in the tibial nerve,[33–37] deep peroneal nerve,[38] and first branch of the lateral plantar nerve.[39] When failure presents, the patient's symptoms may show no improvement, partial improvement, or temporary improvement for a short period of time.[40]

With compression neuropathies, incomplete decompression of the bone or soft tissue that is creating impingement is one of major cause of recurrence. Thus, addressing malunions, bony prominences, bony fragments, fascial or soft tissue impingement, and incomplete releases of previously treated entrapment syndromes should yield a beneficial outcome.[22] However, this will not yield the best results if the integrity of the nerve is compromised.

Revision TTS

When performing revisional nerve surgery in the tarsal tunnel, it is important to perform release of the all nerves of the tarsal tunnel, even if they were not all previously released in the primary surgery. They include the posterior tibial nerve, medial plantar nerve, lateral plantar nerve, and medial calcaneal nerve. The medial and lateral plantar nerves need to be released at the flexor retinaculum fascia of the abductor hallucis. The medial and lateral plantar nerve fascial septum is excised and the medial calcaneal nerve tunnel is released as described by Barker colleagues.[41] Raikin and Mannich[40] identified factors that impact on the success of tarsal tunnel surgery, which include incorrect diagnosis, adhesive neuritis, intraneural damage, and double crush syndrome. Incomplete release of compressive structures or adhesions during the postoperative course can cause symptoms to persist. When performing a revisional neurolyis in the presence of incomplete release, it is important to release the posterior tibial nerve while identifying the point of compression that was unreleased. In the presence of adhesions secondary to the postoperative period, other options to prevent the nerve from being adhered after the revision surgery are discussed with nerve wrapping and grafting.

Numerous reports have shown poor outcomes related to inadequate initial release of patients with TTS.[29,32,40] Poor results with revisional surgery have been seen with patients with radiculopathy or with systemic disease. Revisional surgery has been recommended to avoid surgical decompression in patients with connective tissue disease, as they may have subclinical neuropathy.[40] Kaplan and Kernahan[42] operated on one patient without symptom relief after tarsal tunnel surgery. The revision procedure was extended decompression distally into the sole of the foot, and the patient had complete symptom relief (Evidence-Based Medicine or EBM Level IV). Zeiss and colleagues[43] discovered in reoperation of two patients, after initial tarsal tunnel compression release, that incomplete release of the flexor retinaculum can lead to recurrence of symptoms (EBM Level IV). Eberhard and Millesi[44] operated on two patients who had two, and one patient who had seven, previous surgeries for TTS (EBM Level IV). The procedures used included the removal of the abductor hallucis muscle or its fascia; however, none of the patients experienced relief of their symptoms. Pfeiffer and Cracchiolo[45] operated on six patients with previous tarsal tunnel surgeries. Four had one previous tarsal tunnel operation, one had two, and one had four previous operations. Procedure involved the dissection of the tibial nerve, and the deep abductor hallucis fascia was divided over the medial plantar nerve. Novotny and colleagues[46] found results of 100% with release of posterior tibial nerve and its branches, and coverage with radial free forearm flap (EBM Level V). Zahari[47] also had complete resolution of symptoms after re-exploration of the posterior tibial nerve with release from scar tissue (EBM level V). Skalley colleagues[32] evaluated three groups of revision tarsal tunnel surgery patients. Patients who had no significant scarring and inadequate release of the posterior tibial nerve did much better postoperatively than patients who had scarring with adequate release or patients who had both scarring and inadequate release (EBM Level IV). Gould initially reported the use of the procedure in the foot and ankle with 63% good or excellent results with the vein wrap procedure; however, 25% of patients experienced worsening of their symptoms.[48] Barker and colleagues[41] reported revisional peripheral nerve surgery in 44 patients who had previous tarsal tunnel surgery by performing neurolysis of the posterior tibial nerve, medial plantar nerve, lateral plantar nerve, and calcaneal nerves. The patients had a mean follow-up of 2.2 years and outcome results showed 54% were excellent and 24% were good.

Revisional neuroma excision

In the planning of the revisional plantar neurectomy, a plantar incision is recommended. This will allow tracing of the branch of the common digital nerve off of the medial-plantar or lateral-plantar nerve distally to the site of the stump neuroma formation. This will allow for adequate length of the nerve to resect and bury into the intrinsic musculature of the foot.[49–52]

Some investigators advocate re-exploration of the interspace where the previous surgery was performed.[50,53] Beskin and Baxter evaluated two surgical techniques that were used to resect the nerve over a 2.5-year period, using either the previous dorsal incision or a transverse-plantar incision proximal to the metatarsal heads.[53] Overall results revealed significant improvement for greater than 80% of patients after their final operation (EBM Level IV). Johnson and colleagues[50] re-explored 39 patients with recurrent interdigital neuroma. Of these, 33 patients received a longitudinal plantar incision and four received a dorsal incision (EBM-Level IV). The investigators found 22 patients obtained complete relief or marked improvement in pain. The success rates of these revision surgeries reported higher success rates than previously published studies. Stamatis and Myerson retrospectively reviewed 49 patients, where re-exploration through a dorsal approach and nerve transaction at the proximal site was performed in 60 interspaces for recurrence or persistent symptoms[54] (EBM-Level IV). Based on their study, Stamatis and Myerson found high dissatisfaction rates with their approach for revision surgery similar to other reported re-exploration revision surgeries.

Reported complications associated with primary surgical intervention for neuromas (nerve resection, neurolysis) include but are not limited to dead space hematoma, numbness, stump neuroma, residual pain, contracted digits, and inadequate resection of the nerve.[55] The rates of residual symptoms reported after primary excision for neuroma surgery can be as very high.[56] One of most common complications reported is persistent symptoms after primary excision of interdigital neuroma, where the patient continues to experience the original pain before surgical correction. In a retrospective review of primary resection of interdigital neuromas by Coughlin and colleagues, 26 of 81 patients reported residual pain at final follow-up, along with scar sensitivity, and shoe and activity modification.[55]

Revison superficial peroneal nerve

Chiodo and Miller[6] compared 27 consecutive patients with superficial peroneal neuroma in two different groups: one group with transection and burial of the proximal peroneal nerve stump into muscle and the other group with transection and burial of the proximal stump into bone (EBM level IV). In the group with transection of the superficial peroneal neuroma and burial into muscle, 4 out of 16 patients required revisional surgery because of recurrent neuropathic symptoms. All four had proximal resection with burial into bone. The average perceived relief of pain improving was 79%. These patients had less pain, especially on the skin of the anterolateral leg, but still had some residual deep pain. In the group with transection and burial of proximal stump into bone, no patients required revision surgery because of recurrent neuropathic symptoms.

Diabetic neuropathy

The results of peripheral nerve release are encouraging and rates of revisional surgery have yet to be reported. There are numerous reports published in the literature that show the positive results of using this procedure.[57–61] However, most of the studies that have been published have questionable research designs and are evidence-based level IV studies. Future quality studies (evidence-based level I or II) are needed before this procedure becomes more widely accepted among foot and ankle surgeons.[62] The discussions about the surgical treatment of diabetic peripheral neuropathy has led to an improved understanding and dialog about the treatment of peripheral nerve disorders in diabetic and nondiabetic patients.

Nerve Wrapping

Originally described in the upper extremity, the procedure of nerve wrapping has been expanded for use in the lower-extremity revision nerve surgery.[63] The goal of performing this procedure with revision neurolysis is to provide a barrier, by using an autogenous harvested vein, designed to protect a nerve from external compromise, relieve symptoms, and improve function in patients with adhesive neuralgia.[64] The veins that have been reported are glutalderyhde-preserved umbilical veins in the upper extremity and autogenous saphenous veins.[63,64] Based on a case report, histologic studies after 17 months postoperatively in a patient who underwent this procedure revealed vein graft tissue in direct apposition to the nerve, with no fibrous scarring within or around the nerve.[65] This procedure is commonly performed in conjunction with a neurolysis procedure, which releases the nerve at the site of scarring. Although other forms of protecting the nerve are available, ultimate success of this procedure depends on the integrity of the nerve itself.

Schon and colleagues[63] retrospectively reviewed and found mixed results in patients who were provided revision nerve release with vein wrapping from the saphenous or umbilical vein, for 58 patients who had chronic pain after previous nerve release (EBM Level IV).

Nerve Grafts

Free nerve grafts rely on the formation of adhesions for their survival, which is dependent on in growth of blood vessels from the recipient bed site. Following peripheral nerve release, a normal nerve may regain its mobility by regeneration of the gliding tissue, but this is never the case in re-explored free-nerve grafts. Free-nerve grafts are sensitive to tension and, after a graft procedure, the tension caused by mobilization is concentrated on the proximal stump and the proximal end of the graft, and the distal stump and the distal end of the graft perform minimal compensation.[28] Therefore, when performing nerve grafts, the proximal nerve stump must have enough mobility that it will allow for range of motion of the foot and ankle without creating undue tension on the nerve graft.

Nerve Adjuncts

Many techniques have been employed to alter the local environment, such as fat grafts, muscle flaps, rerouting, and vascularized nerve graft. The aim is to allow the scarred nerve to heal in a new environment free of adhesions.[31] Another adjunct used is nerve stimulation, which provides relief of symptoms by blocking the pain-signal transmission.[66] These procedures may provide relief after all other treatment options have failed. The theory is based on sending nonpainful touch signals to the brain to interfere with pain-signal transmission and prevent the perception of pain.[67]

SUMMARY

Revision peripheral nerve surgery can provide benefits to patients experiencing symptoms after a failed primary procedure. It is important to understand why the initial procedure failed and whether the symptoms are created by internal or external factors. Once the causative factors are identified by the clinical examination, radiologic, and electrodiagnostic studies, many different treatment options exist to provide relief of the patient's symptoms and improve their quality of life. There is a more clear understanding of the clinical signs of peripheral nerve disorders, but diagnosing early peripheral nerve disorders using objective parameters continues to be elusive in a number of patients. Those with documented palpable lesions neighboring peripheral nerves or with MRI findings of a space-occupying lesion are limited in number. In patients with failed primary peripheral nerve surgery, where no clear objective lesions or pathology is present, the best course of action is commonly the more difficult decision, which is to treat them medically and to avoid additional surgery. However, given that most of the literature is supported by fair evidence (EBM Grade B- treatment options are supported by fair evidence consistent with Level III or IV studies), there are many different options available for revision peripheral nerve surgery when it is necessary.

REFERENCES

1. Durlacher L. A treatise on corns, bunions, the disease of nails and the general management of the feet. London: Simpkin, Marshall; 1845.
2. Kay D, Bennett GL. Morton's neuroma. Foot Ankle Clin N Am 2003;8(1):49–59.
3. Medicino SS, Rockett MS. Morton's neuroma: update on diagnosis and imaging. Clin Podiatr Med Surg 1997;14(2):303–11.
4. Weinfeld SB, Myerson MS. Interdigital neuritis: diagnosis and treatment. J Am Acad Orthop Surg 1996;4:328–35.
5. Graham CE, Graham DM. Morton's neuroma: a microscopic evaluation. Foot Ankle 1984;5:150–3.
6. Chiodo CP, Miller SD. Surgical treatment of superficial peroneal neuroma. Foot Ankle 2004;25(10):689–94.
7. Keck C. The tarsal-tunnel syndrome. J Bone Joint Surg 1962;44A:180–2.
8. Lam SJS. A tarsal-tunnel syndrome. Lancet 1962;2:1354–5.
9. Kopell HP, Thompson WAL. Peripheral entrapment neuropathies of the lower extremity. N Engl J Med 1960;262:56–60.
10. Pringle RM, Protheroe K, Mukherjee SK. Entrapment neuropathy of the sural nerve. J Bone Joint Surg Br 1974;56:465–8.
11. Goecker RM, Banks AS. Analysis of release of the 1st branch of lateral plantar nerve. J Am Podiatr Med Assoc 2000;90(6):281–6.

12. Baxter DE, Pfeffer GB. Treatment of chronic heel pain by surgical release of the first branch of the lateral plantar nerve. Clin Orthop Relat Res 1992;279:229–36.
13. Dellon AL. Diabetic neuropathy: review of a surgical approach to restore sensation, relieve pain, and prevent ulceration and amputation. Foot Ankle 2004;25(10): 749–55.
14. Schon LC, Easley ME. Chronic pain. In: Myerson MS, editor. Foot and ankle disorders. Philadelphia: WB Saunders Co.; 2000. p. 851–81.
15. Schon LC, Anderson CD, Easley ME, et al. Surgical treatment of chronic lower extremity neuropathic pain. Clin Orthop Relat Res 2001;389:156–64.
16. Upton AR, McComas AJ. The double crush syndrome in nerve entrapment syndromes. Lancet 1973;2(7825):359–62.
17. Hurst LC, Weissberg D, Carroll RE. The relationship of the double crush to carpal tunnel syndrome (an analysis of 1,000 cases of carpal tunnel syndrome). J Hand Surg [Br] 1985;10:202–4.
18. Majlesi J, Togay H, Unalan H, et al. The sensitivity and specificity of the slump and the straight leg raising tests in patients with lumbar disc herniation. J Clin Rheumatol. 2008;14(2):87–91.
19. Downey MS, Sorrento DL, et al. Tarsal tunnel syndrome. In: Banks AS, Downey MS, Martin DE, editors. McGlamry's Comprehensive Textbook of Foot and Ankle surgery. 3rd Edition. Philadelphia: Williams and Wilkins; 2001. p. 1266–78.
20. Trepman E, Kadel NJ, Chisholm K, et al. Effect of foot and ankle position on tarsal tunnel compartment pressure. Foot Ankle Int 1999;20(11):721–6.
21. Lee DH, Claussen DH, Oh S. Clinical nerve conduction and needle electromyography studies. J Am Acad Orthop Surg 2004;12:276–87.
22. Vora AM, Schon LC. Revision peripheral nerve surgery. Foot Ankle Clin 2004;9(2): 305–18.
23. Budak F, Bamaç B, Ozbek A, et al. Nerve conduction studies of lower extremities in pes planus subjects. Electromyogr Clin Neurophysiol. 2001;41(7):443–6.
24. Bailie DS, Kelikian AS. Tarsal tunnel syndrome: diagnosis, surgical technique, and functional outcome. Foot Ankle Int 1998;19(2):65–72.
25. Abadier AR. Diagnostic nerve blocks. In: Omer, Jr. GE, Spinner M, Van Beek AL, editors. Management of Peripheral Nerve Problems. 2nd Edition. Philadelphia: WB Saunders Co; 1998. p. 65–76.
26. Dellon AL. Management of peripheral nerve problems in the upper and lower extremity using neurosensory testing. Hand Clin. 1999;15:697–715.
27. Grabois M, Puentes J, Lidsky M. Tarsal tunnel syndrome in rheumatoid arthritis. Arch Phys Med Rehabil 1981;62(8):401–3.
28. DiDomenico LA, Masternick EB. Anterior tarsal tunnel syndrome. Clin Podiatr Med Surg 2006;23(3):611–20.
29. Rosson GD, Spinner RJ, Dellon AL. Tarsal tunnel surgery for treatment of tarsal ganglion: a rewarding operation with devastating potential complications. J Am Podiatr Med Assoc 2005;95(5):459–63.
30. Zachary LS, Dellon ES, Nicholas EM, et al. The structural basis of Felice Fontana's spiral bands and their relationship to nerve injury. J Reconstr Microsurg 1993; 9(2):131–8.
31. Abe Y, Doi K, Kawai S. An experimental model of peripheral nerve adhesion in rabbits. Br J Plast Surg 2005;58(4):533–40.
32. Skalley TC, Schon LC, Hinton RY, et al. Clinical results following revision tibial nerve release. Foot Ankle Int 1994;15(7):360–7.
33. Lau JTC, Daniels TR. Tarsal tunnel syndrome: a review of literature. Foot Ankle Int 1999;20:201–9.

34. Turan I, Rivero-Melian C, Guntner P, et al. Tarsal tunnel syndrome: outcome of surgery in longstanding cases. Clin Orthop 1997;343:151–6.
35. Mendicino SS, Mendicino RW. The tarsal tunnel syndrome and its surgical decompression. Clin Podiatr Med Surg 1991;8(3):501–12.
36. Mahan KT, Rock JJ, Hillstrom HJ. Tarsal tunnel syndrome. A retrospective study. J Am Podiatr Med Assoc 1996;86(2):81–91.
37. Sammarco GJ, Chang L. Outcome of surgical treatment of tarsal tunnel syndrome. Foot Ankle Int 2003;24(2):125–31.
38. Gessini L, Jandolo B, Pietrangeli A. The anterior tarsal tunnel syndrome: report of four cases. J Bone Joint Surg Am 1984;66:786–7.
39. Jolly GP, Zgonis T, Hendrix CL. Neurogenic heel pain. Clin Podiatr Med Surg 2005;22(1):101–13.
40. Raikin SM, Minnich JM. Failed tarsal tunnel syndrome surgery. Foot Ankle Clin 2003;8(1):159–74.
41. Barker AR, Rosson GD, Dellon AL. Outcome of neurolysis for failed tarsal tunnel surgery. J Reconstr Microsurg 2008;24(2):111–8.
42. Kaplan PE, Kernahan WT. Tarsal tunnel syndrome. J Bone Joint Surg Am 1981;63:96–9.
43. Zeiss J, Fenton P, Ebraheim N, et al. Magnetic resonance imaging for ineffectual tarsal tunnel surgical treatment. Clin Orthop Relat Res 1991;264:264–6.
44. Eberhard D, Millesi H. Pain syndromes of the tibial nerve at the leg-foot transition. Wien Klin Wochenschr 1993;105:462–6.
45. Pfeiffer WH, Cracchiolo A 3rd. Clinical results after tarsal tunnel decompression. J Bone Joint Surg Am 1994;76(8):1222–30.
46. Novotny DA, Kay DB, Parker MG. Recurrent tarsal tunnel syndrome and the radial forearm free flap. Foot Ankle Int 1996;17:641–3.
47. Zahari DT, Ly P. Recurrent tarsal tunnel syndrome. J Foot Surg 1992;31:385–7.
48. Gould JS. Treatment of the painful injured nerve in-continuity. In: Gelberman GH, editor. Operative Nerve Repair and Reconstruction. Philadelphia: JB Lippincott Co.; 1991. p. 1541–50.
49. Nelms BA, Bishop JO, Tullos HS. Surgical treatment of recurrent Morton's neuroma. Orthopedics 1984;7:1708–11.
50. Johnson JE, Johnson KA, Unni KK. Persistent pain after excision of an interdigital neuroma: results of reoperation. J Bone Joint Surg Am 1988;70-A:651–7.
51. Wolfforth SF, Dellon AL. Treatment of recurrent neuroma of the interdigital nerve by implantation of the proximal nerve into muscle in the arch of the foot. J Foot Ankle Surg 2001;40(6):404–10.
52. Dellon AL. Treatment of recurrent metatarsalgia by neuroma resection and muscle implantation: case report and proposed algorithm of management for Morton's neuroma. Microsurgery 1989;10:256–9.
53. Beskin JL, Baxter DE. Recurrent pain following interdigital neurectomy-a plantar approach. Foot Ankle 1988;9:34–9.
54. Stamatis ED, Myerson MS. Treatment of recurrence of symptoms after excision of an interdigital neuroma. Journal of Bone Joint Surg Br 2004;86-B:48–53.
55. Coughlin MJ, Pinsonneault T. Operative treatment of interdigital neuroma: a long-term follow-up study. J Bone Joint Surg 2001;83:1321–8.
56. Wu KK. Morton's interdigital neuroma: a clinical review of its etiology, treatment, and results. J Foot Ankle Surg 1996;35:112–9.
57. Aszmann OC, Kress KM, Dellon AL. Results of decompression of peripheral nerves in diabetics: a prospective, blinded study. Plast Reconstr Surg 2000;106(4):816–22.

58. Wood WA, Wood MA. Decompression of peripheral nerves for diabetic neuropathy in the lower extremity. J Foot Ankle Surg 2003;42(5):268–75.
59. Rader AJ. Surgical decompression in lower-extremity diabetic peripheral neuropathy. Am Podiatr Med Assoc 2005;95(5):446–50.
60. Valdivia JM, Dellon AL, Weinand ME, et al. Surgical treatment of peripheral neuropathy: outcomes from 100 consecutive decompressions. J Am Podiatr Med Assoc 2005;95(5):451–4.
61. Dellon AL. Diabetic neuropathy: medical and surgical approaches. Clin Podiatr Med Surg 2007;24:425–48.
62. Cain J. Current concepts in surgical management of diabetic neuropathy. Presented at the 66th Annual Scientific Conference of the American College of Foot and Ankle Surgeons; Long Beach (CA), Feb 2008.
63. Schon LC, Lam PWC, Easley ME, et al. Complex salvage procedures for severe lower extremity nerve pain. Clin Orthop Relat Res 2001;391:171–80.
64. Masear VR, Tulloss JR, St. Mary E, et al. Venous wrapping of nerves to prevent scarring. J Hand Surg 1990;15A:817–8, Abstract.
65. Campbell JT, Schon LC, Burkhardt LD. Histopathologic findings in autogenous saphenous vein graft wrapping for recurrent tarsal tunnel syndrome: a case report. Foot Ankle Int 1998;19:766–9.
66. Waisbrod H, Panhans C, Hansen D, et al. Direct nerve stimulation for painful peripheral neuropathies. J Bone Joint Surg 1985;67B:470–2.
67. Gybels J, Van Calenbergh F. The treatment of pain due to peripheral nerve injury by electrical stimulation of the injured nerve. Adv Pain Res Ther 1990;13:217–22.

Complications and Salvage of Elective Central Metatarsal Osteotomies

Richard Derner, DPM, FACFAS[a,*], Andrew J. Meyr, DPM[b]

KEYWORDS

- Central metatarsal osteotomy • Weil osteotomy
- Surgical complication • Floating toe • Arthrosurface
- Metatarsal parabola • Transfer lesion

One of the most important tools at the disposal of a physician is an underlying knowledge of the pathophysiology contributing to a specific patient complaint. The diagnosis of metatarsalgia can occur as the result of a range of potential etiologies and central ray pathologies. In part because of this variety, many different surgical procedures have been described to alleviate this complaint. It is essential for the foot and ankle surgeon to develop not only the correct diagnosis before initiating surgical intervention, but also a complete understanding of the pathology leading to the complaint. Treatment should be directed toward the underlying pathology causing the symptoms that the patient is experiencing. With an appreciation of this concept, the surgeon and the patient can work together in the preoperative phase to develop a mutual understanding of both the specific diagnosis and the expected outcomes of surgical intervention.

This article is written with the defined scope of potential complications that can arise after elective central metatarsal osteotomies. Although the literature is replete with studies examining post-operative outcomes after surgical intervention for metatarsalgia, the bulk of these represent nothing more than extended case series with variable follow-up periods.[1–21] There are no controlled, prospective studies that would provide the level of evidence necessary to compare multiple procedures for the same indication. However, these case series do provide specific complication patterns that appear to be consistent with the indication and irrespective of the specific surgery. The goal of this article is to provide an analysis of these complications as they relate to revisional foot and ankle surgery.

[a] Lake Ridge Foot and Ankle Centers, 1721 Financial Loop, Lake Ridge, VA 22192, USA
[b] INOVA Fairfax Hospital Podiatric Surgical Residency Program, INOVA Fairfax Hospital, Podiatric Surgery Residency Office. T6W, 3300 Gallows Road, Falls Church, VA 20042, USA
* Corresponding author.
E-mail address: richd87@mac.com (R. Derner).

Clin Podiatr Med Surg 26 (2009) 23–35
doi:10.1016/j.cpm.2008.09.003

CLINICAL POINTS OF EMPHASIS

The clinical points of emphasis of this article are for the foot and ankle surgeon to develop a further understanding of the pathoanatomy and pathomechanics leading to specific surgical complications. Based on a review of the extensive case series presented in the medical literature, the authors have a reasonable appreciation of what surgical complications may be anticipated after elective surgical correction of central metatarsal complaints. However, this literature offers very little evidence regarding how to approach these complications in a standardized and logical manner. Instead of studies based on controlled outcome measures, generally only the opinions and specific experiences of the qualified surgeons are presented. Although the authors can unfortunately only offer similar recommendations, it is their goal to additionally emphasize the pathologic etiology of the complication as a basis for treatment intervention. Certainly one cannot hope to surgically correct a complication if they have little understanding as to why it developed.

FLOATING TOE

One of the most common complications after a central metatarsal osteotomy is the development of digital deformities, specifically the floating toe deformity. The floating toe is defined as the inability of a toe to purchase the ground during static stance (**Fig. 1**). It is important to note that in many cases a digital deformity is likely to be present before the initial surgical procedure. In addition to specific anatomic structural causes of lesser metatarsalgia, functional physiologic components also play a large role.[1,17,19,22] Hammertoe contractions with metatarsal–phalangeal joint (MPJ) subluxation/dislocation create a retrograde buckling of the MPJ with a resultant functional plantarflexion of the respective metatarsal.[23] Damage to the MPJ plantar plate additionally exacerbates sagittal plane instability of the joint. Unless the underlying pathology contributing to the metatarsalgia, as well as the soft tissue damage within the MPJ, is addressed during the initial surgical procedure, then postoperative digital complications are nearly inevitable.

In the literature, several articles relate the floating toe to the Weil osteotomy. Migues and colleagues[11] had a 28.5% overall incidence rate and a 50% occurrence rate after Weil osteotomy with proximal interphalangeal joint fusion. In an attempt to prevent this postoperative complication, Beech and colleagues[7] had a 33% incidence of elevated toe despite making their skin incision in the interspace and not directly dorsally.

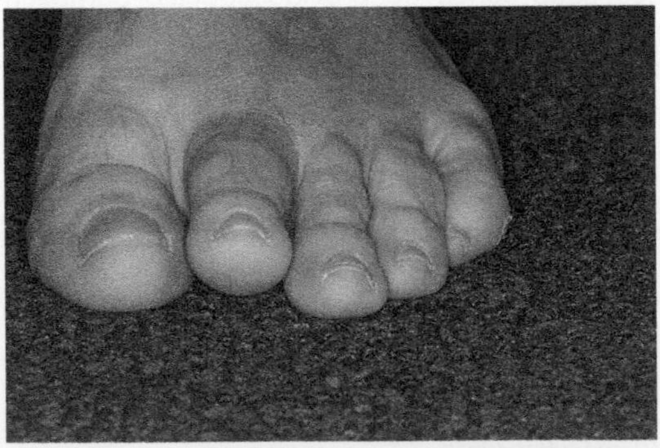

Fig. 1. The clinical appearance of a floating toe deformity after Weil osteotomy and digital arthrodesis.

Further, O'Kane and Kilmartin[5] reported a 20% incidence and Vandeputte and colleagues[14] found a 15% occurrence of floating toe. This is now recognized as a "common complication" when performing the Weil osteotomy.[11]

Several theories attempt to explain the pathomechanics of the floating toe deformity after a central metatarsal osteotomy. Trnka and colleagues[10] specifically investigated the issue of floating toe with the Weil procedure. He performed the osteotomy on cadaveric and sawbones models. Although it is described as being oriented parallel to the weight-bearing surface, Trnka and colleagues found that this was clinically difficult to achieve and that often an unintentional depression of the capital fragment accompanied the intended shortening. In other words, the center of rotation of the MPJ became more proximal and plantar after fixation of the osteotomy. This, in turn, changed the kinematics of the intrinsic musculature balance of the MPJ. Specifically, they concluded that the interosseus muscles now passed dorsal to the MPJ axis and acted as dorsiflexors of the digit as opposed to offering transverse plane stability.[10,11] In addition, it is likely the plantar plate shows a different loading pattern after a metatarsal osteotomy resulting in further sagittal plane instability.

Another theory concerning the cause of floating toe is the relative functional lengthening of the soft tissues around the metatarsophalangeal joint. The primary goal of the Weil osteotomy is to shorten the metatarsal in an attempt to offload plantarly. This shortening creates a slack to all of the tendons of the intrinsic and extrinsic musculature. Anatomically, the extrinsic muscles (extensor digitorum longus and flexor digitorum longus) both send a single slip to each the lesser toes. If a single shortening metatarsal osteotomy is performed, then one slip of the four is relatively lengthened compared with the other digits. This tendon slip then becomes ineffective in both dorsiflexion and specifically plantarflexion. For muscles to function correctly, the tendons must be under proper physiologic tension. This tension is lost when one metatarsal is shortened. A final consideration is the expected scar formation after skin incision. A dorsal skin incision centered over the MPJ can cause a contracture that further exacerbates the floating toe deformity.

As mentioned, specific surgical procedures can lead to the formation of the floating toe. One cannot ignore the overwhelming statistics within the literature. It is possible for this problem to be avoided by taking the proper steps during the initial surgery. Although evidence-based medicine studies are lacking, two specific techniques have been used with some good success either at the time of the initial surgery or in dealing with the postoperative complication.

Initially, it is important to mention that lengthening of the dorsal structures (ie, the extensor tendons) is inadequate when performed alone and should be avoided. Flexor tendon transfers have become a reliable procedure to plantarflex or stabilize the proximal phalanx to the ground (**Fig. 2**). In conjunction with a flexor tendon transfer, a digital arthrodesis must be performed or a reverse hammer toe (hyperextension of the interphalangeal joints) can occur.

A second alternative is the use of a Kirshner wire to maintain the toe in a plantarflexed position postoperatively. This wire is removed approximately 4 to 6 weeks afterward. Temporary stabilization allows for scar tissue to maintain the position of the toe postoperatively. Once the wire is removed, however, it is not unusual to see late elevation of the digit. Therefore, a flexor tendon transfer serves as a better overall option with a higher potential for long term success.

The digital arthrodesis is typically stabilized with a k-wire for fusion and to maintain alignment. Controversy arises for several reasons when the k-wire crosses the metatarsophalangeal joint to stabilize the toe in a plantarflexed position. First, if a wire is placed across the MPJ, arthrosis may occur. This may be from the repeated attempts

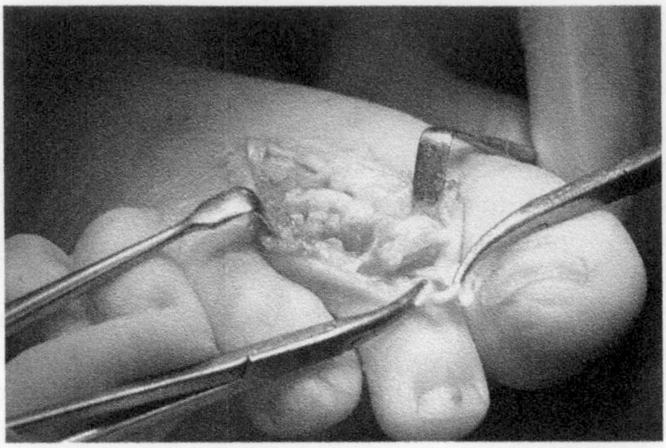

Fig. 2. The lesser digit flexor tendon transfer represents an established adjunctive procedure to prevent the floating toe deformity when performed at the time of initial metatarsal osteotomy.

to splintage with the wire or the lack of motion of this joint for an extended period of time. Additionally, breakage of the pin can occur easily at the pin–metatarsal interface. This often is the case when a patient walks without protective shoe gear with resultant hyperextension or flexion of the joint.

A significant complication may also result when placing a k-wire through a toe into a metatarsal head in which an osteotomy has just been performed. Specifically, a fracture of the metatarsal osteotomy may occur if stress is placed on the toe and is translated along the wire into the metatarsal head. Displacement of the osteotomy occurs and a second surgery is required for realignment.

Hammer toe surgery in conjunction with metatarsal osteotomy increases the incidence of floating toe.[11] For the previously fused toe, treatment consists of the following: extensor tendon lengthening, MPJ capsulotomy, and, most importantly, transfer of the long flexor tendon. However, if an arthroplasty has been performed previously, in addition to the aforementioned, a fusion is attempted. The surgeon is cautioned to be cognizant to minimize further shortening of the toe during a revisional fusion. Placing the digit in a slightly plantarflexed position at the proximal interphalangeal joint for fusion in conjunction with the flexor tendon transfer will help resolve the floating toe.

METATARSAL–PHALANGEAL JOINT STIFFNESS AND POSTTRAUMATIC ARTHRITIS

In addition to the floating toe deformity, the new mechanics of the MPJ after metatarsal osteotomy may result in decreased range of motion and stiffness of the joint. This is again often a consequence of an imposed intrinsic muscular imbalance but may also be the result of a concomitant condition. The surgeon should be aware of existing intra-articular pathology that may be associated with metatarsalgia at the time of the initial procedure. Degenerative joint disease, posttraumatic arthritis, soft tissue adaptive adhesions, Freiberg's infarction, and other conditions may contribute to articular symptoms but will not be resolved with a shortening osteotomy.[1,17,18]

In the past, arthrosis after metatarsal osteotomy has been treated with implant arthroplasty, partial metatarsal head resection, complete metatarsal head resection, or even fusion of the MPJ. Cobalt chrome hemi implants, inserted either into the base of the proximal phalanx or to the head of the lesser metatarsal, have shown some promise as a potential treatment alternative. In specific cases the authors have used the Arthrosurface® (Arthrosurface, Franklin, MD) implant to replace the arthritic head of a lesser MPJ (**Fig. 3**). The Arthrosurface is a two-piece device with

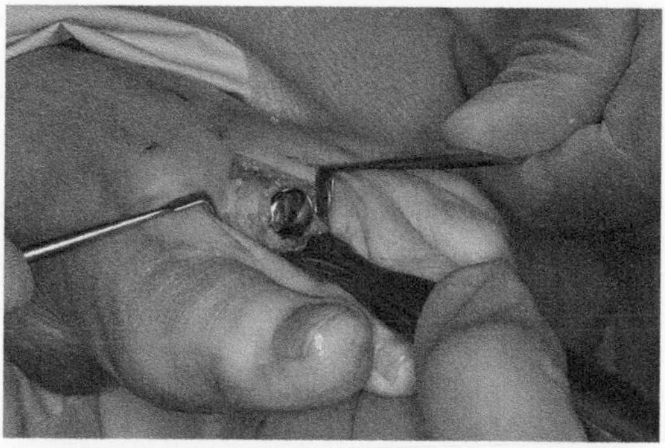

Fig. 3. The final result of a proximal hemi-arthroplasty implant of the second metatarsal-phalangeal joint for posttraumatic arthritis.

a Cobalt chrome articular cap and fixation component. The fixation component is a titanium screw, which is inserted into the head of the metatarsal. Once the exact measurement has been determined, the cap is impacted into the fixation component.

Currently and most commonly, the second metatarsal has been replaced. This implant appears to articulate well with the proximal phalanx base and provides more than adequate motion. Studies are needed to determine its long-term efficacy, but early results in the authors' experience are promising.

TRANSFER LESIONS AND RECURRENCE

The development of transfer lesions after central metatarsal osteotomies probably occurs by the same mechanism as the development of the initial metatarsalgia. The same could be said for the progression of recurrence in the postoperative phase. This is an area in which it appears as though surgeons tend to concentrate more on the art rather than the science of surgery. To develop a full understanding of this complication, it is necessary to take a hard, introspective look at our preoperative evaluation of metatarsalgia as well as the traditional expected outcomes of surgical intervention.

It is intuitive that metatarsalgia develops as the result of an overloaded metatarsal at the MPJ level. Statically, this could result from a structural deformity when a given metatarsal is elongated, is plantarly displaced, or possesses enlarged anatomy (head and condyle) relative to the adjacent metatarsals.[1,17,18] The key is the term "relative." We tend to think of the metatarsals acting as a unit during weight-bearing and gait and assume that a "normal" metatarsal "parabola" will result in the effective transfer of pressure medially and distally during propulsion. An elongated, plantarly displaced or enlarged metatarsal ineffectively increases the pressure on that metatarsal, just as a shortened or dorsally displaced metatarsal decreases the pressure on that metatarsal and subsequently increases the pressure on the adjacent metatarsals.

Using this diagnostic paradigm, the goal of surgical intervention is to recreate a normal metatarsal parabola. Preoperatively this is most commonly evaluated with static plain film radiographs. The relative metatarsal parabola, protrusion, or length pattern is determined with a dorsoplantar view in the angle and base of gait. However, it is important to note that this view only gives information about the transverse plane position of the metatarsals and how far distally they extend relative to each other in the stance phase of gait. It does not give the surgeon information regarding the relative sagittal or frontal plane position of the metatarsals or information about the transverse plane positions during propulsion when symptoms are most likely to occur. Because of the metatarsal declination angles, it is instinctive that as the metatarsals extend distally they also extend plantarly, but this cannot be fully evaluated with just a dorsoplantar view.

It is also frustrating but important to consider that we don't exactly know what "normal" is for transverse plane distal extension of the metatarsals.[17,24] Both relative and absolute measurements have been proposed. With respect to relative measurements, traditionally a gradual taper is expected to progress from the second to the fifth metatarsal, with the first metatarsal being somewhat shorter than the second (2 >1= 3 >4 >5), although arguments have also been proposed that the first and second metatarsals should be of the same length (1= 2 > 3 > 4 > 5).[22,25–29] Tangential measurements can be drawn to evaluate the taper of the lesser metatarsals (**Fig. 4**).[30] However, the obvious limitation of these measurements is the assumption that the two reference points (distal aspects of two lesser metatarsals) are normal. Absolute measurements can be derived from the variation off tangential lines and also through the classic system proposed by Hardy and Clapham in 1951 (see **Fig. 4**).[31] These give the surgeon a quantified goal for transverse plane surgical correction that can be approximated intraoperatively.

Sesamoid axial and other radiographic projections traditionally are used to evaluate the position of the metatarsals with respect to the sagittal and frontal planes.[32,33] Although the dorsoplantar projection provides information regarding the relative "length" of the metatarsals in the transverse plane, these views provide the relative "height" of the metatarsals from the weight-bearing surface.

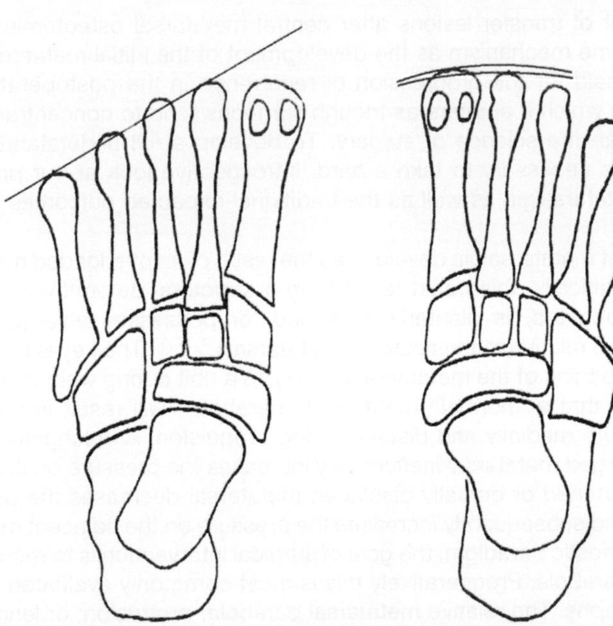

Fig. 4. The left foot in this figure shows how a tangential measurement can be used to relatively quantify the expected lesser metatarsal parabola taper. An absolute measurement between two adjacent metatarsals can be determined using the method described first by Hardy and Clapham (right foot in the figure).

We assume that the static stance position of the metatarsal heads (which is the position these radiographs are taken in) should be equal in terms of "height" from the weight-bearing surface. These views, however, do not take into account the functional components of the metatarsal heads during propulsion and are not a true measure of sagittal plane position.

Therefore, surgeons are cautioned against an over reliance on radiographs during the evaluation of metatarsalgia and should not blindly "treat the x-ray." For one, these measurements are highly dependent on foot and radiograph position. Small changes in the foot position or beam projection can significantly change the presentation of the metatarsal parabola image. Unfortunately, many limitations and unanswered questions remain with respect to our current understanding of distal metatarsal anatomy, function, and pathomechanics and the development of metatarsalgia, recurrence, and transfer lesions:

- *Do static radiographic evaluations provide a valid representation of functional distal metatarsal mechanics?* Metatarsalgia is a functional problem that can be affected by metatarsal hypermobility, retrograde digital buckling, and intra-articular pathologies in addition to static structural abnormalities.[17] Plain film radiographs do not take into account these functional variables or a measure of structural anatomy during the propulsive phase of gait. Particularly in the setting of recurrence and transfer lesions, functional pedobarographic studies should be considered to provide the surgeon with a fuller picture of the scope of the pathology.[14,34–37]
- *What is the correlation between structural abnormality and clinical symptoms?* At this time we do not have outcome-based evidence that correlates quantitative measurements to qualitative complaints. It is unknown if shortening a metatarsal with a Weil osteotomy by 5 mm will have any more or less effect than shortening it by 2.5 mm in a given situation. We also do not know if altering the metatarsal declination angle with a proximal wedge osteotomy by 5° as opposed to 15° will have more or less of a functional difference.
- *Does the relative metatarsal length and divergence from a tapered parabola lead to symptoms, or is the relative metatarsal height more clinically relevant?* An answer to this question may change potential treatment interventions. We do not know the functional difference between osteotomies that have a greater effect on metatarsal length (e.g., Weil osteotomies, proximal oblique osteotomies, diaphyseal step-down osteotomies) versus those that have a greater effect on metatarsal height (e.g., osteoclasis, V osteotomies, wedge resections).

Another possible consideration in the setting of both recurrent and transfer lesions is that of ankle equinus. Although preoperative evaluation of metatarsalgia generally is focused on the structural osseous anatomy of the distal metatarsals and the soft tissue anatomy of the metatarsal-phalangeal joints, this does not rule out the involvement of other pathologic forces. Interestingly, much of what we know about this facet of metatarsalgia is inferred from research on diabetic foot ulcerations and not from this specific complaint. Equinus has not traditionally been described as a contributing pathologic force in the development of forefoot complaints.[38–40] However, the triad of neuropathy, ischemia, and trauma is well established with regard to the development of forefoot submetatarsal diabetic ulcerations.[41–44] In addition to structural osseous and soft tissue abnormalities leading to increased forefoot pressures, the contribution of ankle equinus as a cause of forefoot trauma has been the focus of intervention.[45–54]

In fact, gastrocnemius recession and tendo-Achilles lengthening have been described as primary surgical interventions in the treatment of diabetic forefoot ulcerations in addition to treatment with local wound care.[45–54] Studies have found significantly decreased quantitative forefoot pressure measurements after these procedures. Diabetic wounds heal at faster rates, and recurrence levels are lower when these techniques are used to remove one component of the underlying pathology.[45–54] Certainly increased forefoot pressure contributes to the complaint of metatarsalgia, but further study is required to determine what role ankle equinus plays in this force. It should at least be considered in the setting of recurrent forefoot surgical complications.

Transfer lesions occur as a result of overcorrection of a metatarsal problem. However, ignoring some simple preoperative findings may prevent this problem postoperatively. Despite pain under one specific metatarsal head, if shortening is indicated, evaluation of overall metatarsal length is crucial in preventing transfer lesions. One must consider shortening two or three metatarsals at the same setting to prevent returning to the operating room in the future. This is obvious where the second and third metatarsals are long compared with the fourth metatarsal. One should consider shortening both metatarsals in this situation, and not only one metatarsal. Although this will not guarantee a perfect outcome, it does give the patient the best opportunity for success.

When treating the transfer lesions, one needs to assess the extent of elevation of the metatarsal already surgically addressed. If elevation is severe, surgery should include plantarflexion of this metatarsal and possibly elevation of the adjacent metatarsal. Plantarflexion of the metatarsal is performed either by a V-type osteotomy or oblique sliding osteotomy if both length and plantarflexion are needed. Callus distraction is rarely required to elongate a shortened metatarsal but can be used if necessary.

Undercorrection is also a very challenging problem to prevent in central metatarsal surgery. How much elevation is enough is difficult to ascertain preoperatively by any known scientific measurement. Therefore, the surgeon must "guess" as to the appropriate amount of elevation and shortening. "Feel" becomes most important in determining the correct length and elevation. The end result of an undercorrected elevational osteotomy is usually additional elevation at a second setting. It is also not unusual to see stress fractures at the surgical site postoperatively if undercorrection had occurred (**Fig. 5**).

Treatment of a cavus foot structure with metatarsalgia must be looked at globally. Specifically, elevating one or even two metatarsals is not enough to resolve the cavus foot problem; therefore, all metatarsals including the first and fifth may need to be elevated. The cavus foot is a very complex problem with distal migration of the fat pad, hammertoe deformities, and midfoot/rearfoot abnormalities all contributing to lesser metatarsalgia. It is not unusual to see patients with postoperative problems after single hammertoe repair and metatarsal osteotomy with a cavus foot. This

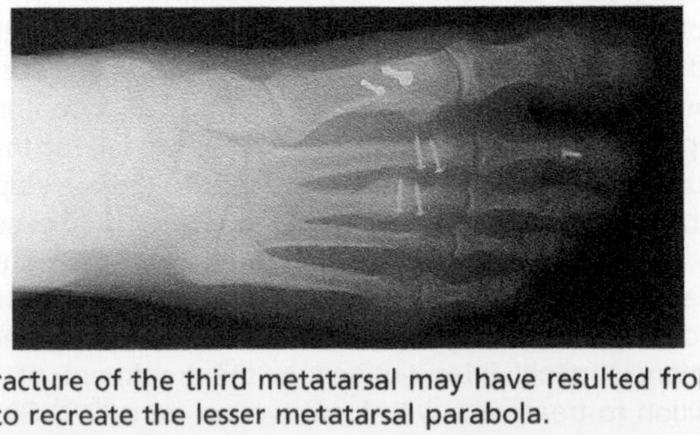

Fig. 5. This stress fracture of the third metatarsal may have resulted from undercorrection while attempting to recreate the lesser metatarsal parabola.

occurrence is, unfortunately, too common, with the surgeon ignoring the entire foot and only addressing the one complaint. Transfer lesions are inevitable, and the surgeon must address the entire foot structure in an attempt to treat the cavus foot.

MALUNION AND NONUNION

Malunion and malposition as a complication of elective central metatarsal osteotomies are usually the result of intraoperative surgeon error, inadequate hardware, or hardware failure. Very few studies have specifically examined the effect of fixation on the outcome of lesser metatarsal surgery,[55,56] and even fewer clinical conclusions can be drawn from this literature. Despite this, some general considerations should be appreciated. The structural anatomy of the lesser metatarsals is orientated such that the loading force is transmitted in a dorsal direction through the metatarsal head. With weight bearing the metatarsals contribute to the longitudinal arches of foot with tension forces plantarly and compressive forces dorsally. This allows for a relatively intrinsic stability with certain osteotomies such as the distal oblique type and proximal dorsal wedges. However, other types of osteotomies are more susceptible to these forces such as the distal V and step-down types.

Delayed or nonunion of metatarsal osteotomies can occur if the vascular anatomy is not appreciated during the initial surgery or if the patient is not appropriately offloaded in the postoperative phase. Nutrient arteries supplying the lesser metatarsals arise from the plantar metatarsal arteries and generally enter the diaphyseal portion of the metatarsal from the protected side.[57] Distally, the plantar metatarsal artery also gives another distinct branch at the level of the metaphyseal–diaphyseal junction directly supplying the metatarsal head and capsular aspects of the plantar plate. The plantar capsular branches anastomose in a well-defined network about the metatarsal head with dorsal capsular branches supplied by the dorsal metatarsal arteries. The dorsal metatarsal arteries are usually distinct branches of the arcuate artery and travel in the intermetatarsal space within the substance of the respective dorsal interosseous muscles.[17,58–60]

Most studies have noted a very successful fusion rate for the Weil osteotomy.[1–4,6,7,14,19] No other studies have been performed for fusion rates on the many other types of lesser metatarsal osteotomies. One would think that this shows the low rate of nonunions in central metatarsal surgery.

By the authors' experience, a nonunion can occur with the offset-V osteotomy but has not been seen with either the Weil or proximal oblique osteotomy (**Fig. 6**). In performing the offset-V technique, a guide pin is placed from dorsal to plantar as an axis guide at the apex of the osteotomy. This wire is placed off center within the metatarsal head to create a long and short wing. This allows for screw fixation of the osteotomy. In addition to elevation, shortening is produced by removing a small piece of bone from the side of the osteotomy. If the apex is too proximal, the osteotomy is made solely within diaphyseal bone, leading to slow bone healing. Inadequate irrigation resulting in excessive heat to the diaphyseal bone may cause osteonecrosis and ultimately lead to a nonunion. Finally, early weight bearing can cause failure of the fixation and instability at the osteotomy site resulting in a nonunion.

Treatment is standard as with any nonunion. Hypertrophic nonunions are stabilized with proper fixation as necessary. Exuberant bone is resected, and, if required, the metatarsal bone is realigned into its proper position. Atrophic nonunions, on the other hand, require hardware removal and resection of necrotic or nonviable bone. Graft is used to maintain length and alignment with fixation to create stability and allow for bone healing. Plate fixation often is used in this setting.

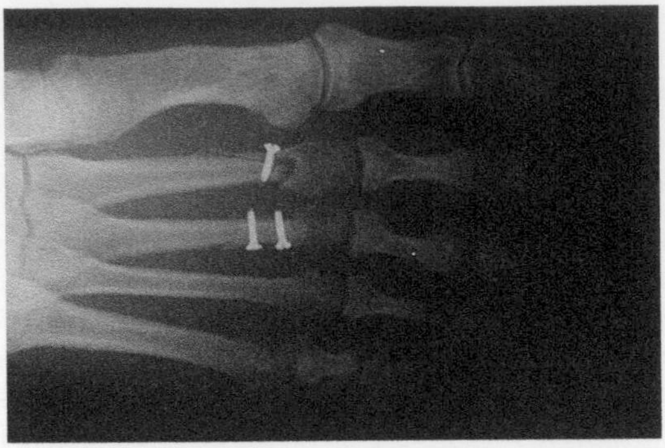

Fig. 6. Nonunion after second metatarsal osteotomy. Note that the osteotomy was performed within the diaphyseal portion of the bone and that only one point of fixation was used.

Postoperatively, the patients are kept non–weight bearing for approximately 2 weeks in a slipper cast or removable cast. This period is followed by partial to full weight bearing with a removable cast with a Plastizote® (Apex, Inc., Teaneck, NJ) cutout to offload the specific metatarsal. At 4 weeks, x-rays are taken with the patient then slowly transitioning to a running-type shoe. Patients undergoing a Weil osteotomy bear weight sooner because of the intrinsic stability of the osteotomy. Smokers and offset-V osteotomy patients are slower in returning to full weight bearing to prevent fracture and delayed/nonunions.

SUMMARY

The goal of this brief review is not only to provide the authors' experiences and potential solutions to surgical complications after elective central metatarsal osteotomies but also a clearer definition of the problem. To avoid postoperative complications, central metatarsal surgery requires precise diagnosis of the patient's complaint and pathology. The surgeon and the patient should work together in the preoperative period to develop a mutual understanding of the expected outcomes of surgical intervention. Additionally, the impetus is on our profession to continue evidence-based outcome research to further our understanding of the many unanswered questions that remain with respect to this topic.

REFERENCES

1. Hofstaetter SG, Hofstaetter JG, Petroutsas JA, et al. The Weil osteotomy: a seven-year follow-up. J Bone Joint Surg Br 2005;87(11):1507–11.
2. Kennedy JG, Deland JT. Resolution of metatarsalgia following oblique osteotomy. Clin Orthop Relat Res 2006;453:309–13.
3. Idusuyi OB, Kitaoka HB, Patzer GL. Oblique metatarsal osteotomy for intractable plantar keratosis: 10-year follow up. Foot Ankle Int 1998;19(6):351–5.
4. Trnka HJ, Mühlbauer M, Zettl R, et al. Comparison of the results of the Weil and Helal osteotomies for the treatment of metatarsalgia secondary to dislocation of the lesser metatarsophalangeal joint. Foot Ankle Int 1999;20(2):72–9.
5. O'Kane C, Kilmartin TE. The surgical management of central metatarsalgia. Foot Ankle Int 2002;23(5):415–9.

6. Cheng YM, Lin SY, Wu CK. Oblique sliding metatarsal osteotomy for pressure metatarsalgia. Gaoxiong Yi Ke Xue Za Zhi 1992;8(8):403–11.
7. Beech I, Rees S, Tagoe M. A retrospective review of the Weil metatarsal osteotomy for lesser metatarsal deformities: an intermediate follow-up analysis. J Foot Ankle Surg 2005;44(5):358–64.
8. Okuda R, Kinoshita M, Morikawa J, et al. Proximal metatarsal osteotomy: relation between 1- to greater than 3-years results. Clin Orthop Relat Res 2005;435:191–6.
9. Khalafi A, Landsman AS, Lautenschlager EP, et al. Plantar forefoot changes after second metatarsal neck osteotomy. Foot Ankle Int 2005;26(7):550–5.
10. Trnka HJ, Nyska M, Parks BG, et al. Dorsiflexion contracture after the Weil osteotomy: results of cadaver study and three-dimensional analysis. Foot Ankle Int 2001;22(1):47–50.
11. Migues A, Slullitel G, Bilbao F, et al. Floating-toe deformity as a complication of the Weil osteotomy. Foot Ankle Int 2004;25(9):609–13.
12. Schwartz N, Williams JE Jr, Marcinko DE. Double oblique lesser metatarsal osteotomy. J Am Podiatry Assoc 1983;73(4):218–20.
13. Lauf E, Weinraub GM. Asymmetric "V" osteotomy: a predictable surgical approach for chronic central metatarsalgia. J Foot Ankle Surg 1996;35(6):550–9.
14. Vandeputte G, Dereymaeker G, Steenwerckx A, et al. The Weil osteotomy of the lesser metatarsals: a clinical and pedobarographic follow-up study. Foot Ankle Int 2000;21(5):370–4.
15. Hatcher RM, Gollier WL, Weil LS. Intractable plantar keratoses: a review of surgical corrections. J Am Podiatr Med Assoc 1978;68:377–86.
16. Pontious J, Lane GD, Moritz JC, et al. Lesser metatarsal V-osteotomy for chronic intractable plantar keratosis. Retrospective analysis of 40 procedures. J Am Podiatr Med Assoc 1998;88(7):323–31.
17. Roukis TS. Central metatarsal head-neck osteotomies: indications and operative techniques. Clin Podiatr Med Surg 2005;22(2):197–222.
18. Jimenez AL, Fishco WD. Part 3: Central metatarsals. In: Banks AS, Downey MS, Martin DE, Miller SJ, editors. McGlamry's comprehensive textbook of foot and ankle surgery. Philadelphia: Lippincott, Williams and Wilkins; 2001. p. 322–38.
19. Barouk LS. Weil's metatarsal osteotomy in the treatment of metatarsalgia. Orthopade 1996;25(4):338–44.
20. Dockery GL. Evaluation and treatment of metatarsalgia and keratotic disorders. In: Myerson MS, editor. Foot and ankle disorders. Philadelphia: W.B. Saunders Company; 2000. p. 359–78.
21. Baravarian B. Lesser metatarsal osteotomy. In: Chang TJ, editor. Master techniques in podiatric surgery: the foot and ankle. Philadelphia: Lippincott, Williams and Wilkins; 2005. p. 85–92.
22. Viladot A. Metatarsalgia due to biomechanical alterations of the forefoot. Orthop Clin North Am 1973;4(1):165–78.
23. Yu GV, Judge MS, Hudson JR, et al. Predislocation syndrome. Progressive subluxation/dislocation of the lesser metarsophalangeal joint. J Am Podiatr Med Assoc 2002;92(4):182–99.
24. Griffin NL, Richmond BG. Cross-sectional geometry of the human forefoot. Bone 2005;37(2):253–6.
25. Dominguez G, Munuera PV, Lafuente G. Relative metatarsal protrusion in the adult: a preliminary study. J Am Podiatr Assoc 2006;96(3):238–44.
26. Sanner WH. Foot segmental relationships and bone morphology. In: Christman RA, editor. Foot and ankle radiology. St. Louis: Churchill Livingstone; 2003. p. 272–302.

27. Bojsen-Møller F. Normal and pathologic anatomy of metatarsals. Orthopade 1982;11(4):148–53.
28. Barouk LS. Metatarsalgia: metatarsal excess of length in dorso-plantar x-ray view in standing position. In: Barouk LS, editor. Forefoot reconstruction. Paris: Springer-Verlag; 2003. p. 214–6.
29. Maestro M, Besse JL, Ragusa M, et al. Forefoot morphotype study and planning method for forefoot osteotomy. Foot Ankle Clin 2003;8(4):695–710.
30. Valley BA, Reese HW. Guidelines for reconstructing the metatarsal parabola with the shortening osteotomy. J Am Podiatr Med Assoc 1991;81(8): 406–13.
31. Hardy RH, Clapham JC. Observations on hallux valgus. based on a controlled series. J Bone Joint Surg Br 1951;33-B(3):376–91.
32. Baron RL, Strugielski CF, Christman RA. Positioning techniques and terminology. In: Christman RA, editor. Foot and Ankle Radiology. St. Louis: Churchill Livingstone; 2003. p. 44–73.
33. Dreeben S, Thomas PB, Noble PC, et al. A new method for radiography of weight-bearing metatarsal heads. Clin Orthop Relat Res 1987;(224):260–7.
34. Snyder J, Owen J, Wayne J, et al. Plantar pressure and load in cadaveric feet after a Weil or Chevron osteotomy. Foot Ankle Int 2005;26(2):158–65.
35. Khalafi A, Landsman AS, Lautenschlager EP, et al. Plantar forefoot pressure changes after second metatarsal neck osteotomy. Foot Ankle Int 2005;26(7): 550–5.
36. Grimes J, Coughlin M. Geometric analysis of the Weil osteotomy. Foot Ankle Int 2006;27(11):985–92.
37. Lau JT, Stamatis ED, Parks BG, et al. Modifications of the Weil osteotomy have no effect on plantar pressure. Clin Orthop Relat Res 2004;(421):194–8.
38. Barrett SL, Jarvis J. Equinus deformity as a factor in forefoot nerve entrapment: treatment with endoscopic gastrocnemius recession. J Am Podiatr Med Assoc 2005;95(5):464–8.
39. DiGiovanni CW, Kuo R, Tejwani N, et al. Isolated gastrocnemius tightness. J Bone Joint Surg Am 2002;84-A(6):962–70.
40. Hill RS. Ankle equinus. Prevalence and linkage to common foot pathology. J Am Podiatr Med Assoc 1995;85(6):295–300.
41. Lavery LA, Armstrong DG, Wunderlich RP, et al. Diabetic foot syndrome: evaluating the prevalence and incidence of foot pathology in Mexican Americans and non-Hispanic whites from a diabetes disease management cohort. Diabetes Care 2003;26(5):1435–8.
42. Laing P. The development and complications of diabetic foot ulcers. Am J Surg 1998;176(2A Suppl):11S–9S.
43. Murray HJ, Boulton AJ. The pathophysiology of diabetic foot ulceration. Clin Podiatr Med Surg 1995;12(1):1–17.
44. Brem H, Sheehan P, Rosenberg HJ, et al. Evidence-based protocol for diabetic foot ulcers. Plastics Recon Surg 2006;117(7S):193S–209S.
45. Van Gils CC, Roeder B. The effect of ankle equines upon the diabetic foot. Clin Podiatr Med Surg 2002;19(3):391–409.
46. Lin SS, Lee TH, Wapner KL. Plantar forefoot ulceration with equinus deformity of the ankle in diabetic patients: the effect of tendo-Achilles lengthening and total contact casting. Orthopedics 1996;19(5):465–75.
47. Lavery LA, Armstrong DG, Boulton AJ. Ankle equinus deformity and its relationship to high plantar pressure in a large population with diabetes mellitus. J Am Podiatr Med Assoc 2002;92(9):479–82.

48. Willrich A, Angirasa AK, Sage RA. Percutaneous tendo Achillis lengthening to promote healing of diabetic plantar foot ulceration. J Am Podiatr Med Assoc 2005;95(3):281–4.
49. Orendurff MS, Rohr ES, Sangeorzan BJ, et al. An equinus deformity of the ankle accounts for only a small amount of the increased forefoot plantar pressure in patients with diabetes. J Bone Joint Surg Br 2006;88(1):65–8.
50. Armstrong DG, Stacpoole-Shea S, Nguyen H, et al. Lengthening of the Achilles tendon in diabetic patients who are at high risk for ulceration of the foot. J Bone Joint Surg Am 1999;81(4):535–8.
51. Holstein P, Lohmann M, Bitsch M, et al. Achilles tendon lengthening, the panacea for plantar forefoot ulceration? Diabetes Metab Res Rev 2004;20(Suppl 1): S37–40.
52. Maluf KS, Meuller MJ, Strube MJ, et al. Tendon Achilles lengthening for the treatment of neuropathic ulcers causes a temporary reduction in forefoot pressure associated with changes in plantar flexor power rather than ankle motion during gait. J Biomech 2004;37(6):897–906.
53. Mueller MJ, Sinacore DR, Hastings MK, et al. Effect of Achilles tendon lengthening on neuropathic plantar ulcers. A randomized clinical trial. J Bone Joint Surg Am 2003;5-A(8):1436–45.
54. Nubé VL, Molyneaux L, Yue DK. Biomechanical risk factors associated with neuropathic ulceration of the hallux in people with diabetes mellitus. J Am Podiatr Med Assoc 2006;96(3):189–97.
55. Jex CT, Wan CJ, Rundell S, et al. Analysis of three types of fixation of the Weil osteotomy. J Foot Ankle Surg 2006;45(1):13–9.
56. Slovenkai MP, Linehan D, McGrady L, et al. Comparison of two fixation methods of oblique lesser metatarsal osteotomies: a biomechanical study. Foot Ankle Int 1995;16(7):437–9.
57. Sarrafian SK. Angiology. In: Anatomy of the foot and ankle. Philadelphia: J.B. Lippincott Company; 1983. p. 261–312.
58. Jaworek TE. Intrinsic vascular alterations within osseous tissue of the lesser metatarsals. Arch Podiatr Med Foot Surg 1978;5(2):9–22.
59. Leemrijse T, Valtin B, Oberlin C. Vascularization of the heads of the three central metatarsals: an anatomical study, its application and considerations with respect to horizontal osteotomies at the neck of the metatarsals. Foot Ankle Surg 1998;4: 57–62.
60. Petersen WJ, Lankes JM, Paulsen F, et al. The arterial supply of the lesser metatarsal heads: a vascular injection study in human cadavers. Foot Ankle Int 2002; 23(6):491–5.

Revision Surgery of the First Ray

Glenn M. Weinraub, DPM, FACFAS[a,*], Ottoniel Mejia, DPM[b]

KEYWORDS

• Revision • First metatarsal • Lapidus
• Arthrodesis • First ray

Every practicing surgeon experiences complications in his or her practice. Inevitably, disruption of the skin and subsequent dissection of soft tissue can lead to infection, hematoma, painful scar formation, and subsequent nerve entrapment. Surgeons who deal with bone have additional complications associated with bone healing. Such complications include nonunions, avascular necrosis, osteotomy dislocations, and painful hardware. The foot and ankle surgeon must have a good understanding of the biomechanics and biology of bone healing and be acquainted with the principles of internal fixation to decrease postoperative complications associated with surgical procedures.[1]

When dealing with the first ray, and in particular when preparing for hallux abductovalgus surgery, numerous guidelines are available to help decide what procedure is most appropriate for the pathology based on radiographic findings. However, these guidelines are not as black and white as some physicians may think. Numerous factors affect the selection of a procedure, including physician preference, physician comfort with a procedure, experience with a procedure, and surgical skills. Various osteotomies exist that aid the physician in addressing first ray pathology.[2]

Hallux abductovalgus can be addressed using various techniques. The pathology is the result of retrograde forces causing an increase in the first intermetatarsal angle. Soft tissue attachments at the lateral base of the proximal phalanx cause adductovarus deformity. The goal of surgery is to reduce the intermetatarsal angle and reduce the forces deforming soft tissue. Various procedures allow reduction of the intermetatarsal angle. The most common procedure is the Austin osteotomy with any one of its numerous modifications.[3] The purist would say that this does not really address the underlying deformity of the increased intermetatarsal angle because the deformity is not addressed at the center of the rotational axis. However the decreased morbidity and the ability to bear weight during recovery makes it pleasing to the surgeon and patient alike. The Lapidus bunionectomy better addresses the root cause of the

[a] Kaiser Permanente Medical Group, Department of Orthopaedic Surgery, Hayward/Fremont, CA 24153, USA
[b] University of California Los Angeles Podiatry Group, 100 UCLA Medical Plaza Suite 460, Los Angeles, CA 90095, USA
* Corresponding author.
E-mail address: gweinraub@aol.com (G.M. Weinraub).

Clin Podiatr Med Surg 26 (2009) 37–45
doi:10.1016/j.cpm.2008.10.001 podiatric.theclinics.com

deformity. However, such a procedure may be challenging for some physicians, especially considering the associated limitations on weight bearing for the patient.[4]

Inherent complications associated with Lapidus bunionectomy include those associated with all surgical procedures, such as infection and hematoma formation. Also however, Lapidus bunionectomy is associated with complications peculiar to this particular procedure. These include recurrent hallux valgus, hallux varus, avascular necrosis, dislocation of the capital fragment, development of painful arthrofibrosis, and pain associated with hardware. With Lapidus bunionectomy, we may worry about nonunion, undercorrection, and excessive shortening of the first ray. The big question remains: For any one specific case of hallux abductovalgus deformity, which of these procedures—Austin osteotomy or Lapidus bunionectomy—is best? Regardless, the saying that "good surgical judgment comes from experience and experience comes from poor surgical judgment" is quite apropos in this setting. This article takes a clinical look at a number of complications related to surgery and trauma of the first ray, and presents a critical discussion of the thought process used to address the complication.

CASE 1

Case 1 involves a 29-year-old physical therapist who underwent an Austin bunionectomy 2 years before presentation. The index procedure was complicated by avascular necrosis of the capital fragment with significant joint collapse. The treating surgeon chose to address this via a total silastic implant. The patient presented complaining of a shortened hallux in extensus and pain under the second metatarsal head (**Fig. 1**).

Analysis of the deformity showed an oversized implant with a short first ray in combination with relative elongation of the second ray. Reestablishment of a normal weight-bearing parabola was paramount in this case. Clearly the second ray needed to be shortened relative to the third ray and the proposed first ray. The dilemma here was how to best address the first ray. Certainly the surgeon could remove the implant and perform an elongating intercalary grafting procedure. However, with removal of the implant, the remaining bone content would be less than optimal to obtain graft stability and hence fusion. Therefore, it was decided to remove the implant and to bone-graft the large primary defect in the hope that a staged fusion procedure could be performed after the first metatarsal had been elongated via distraction osteogenesis (**Fig. 2**).

In this particular case, once the first ray had been brought out to length, the patient opted to delay the proposed plan of docking the distraction segment to the base of the

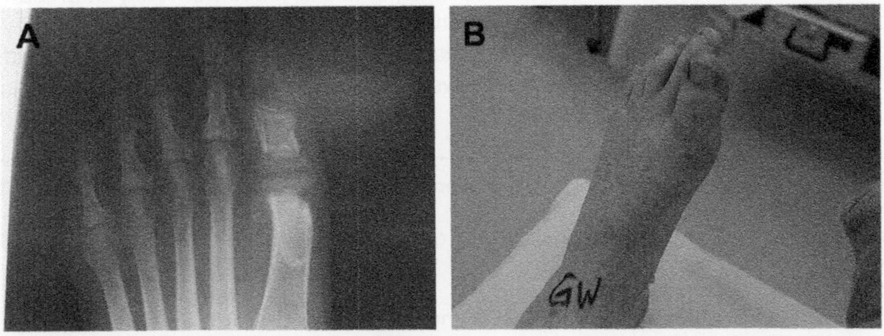

Fig. 1. (*A*) Anterioposterior radiograph from case 1 showing retained silastic total implant at first metatarsophalangeal joint. (*B*) Clinical picture of resultant shortened hallux in extension attitude.

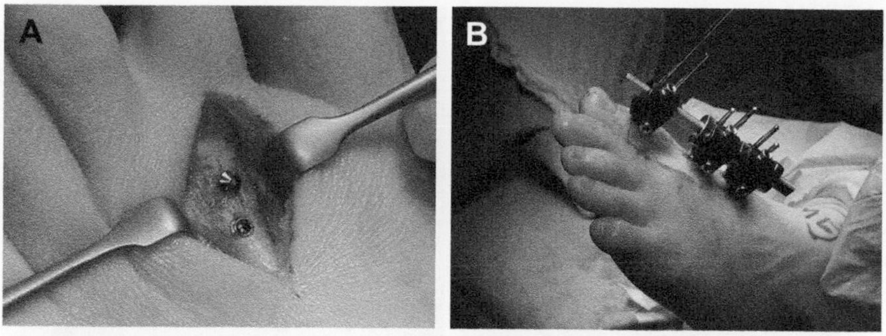

Fig. 2. (*A*) Intraoperative photograph from case 1 of second metatarsal shortening osteotomy in attempt to improve weight-bearing parabola. (*B*) Application of external fixation to both perform distraction osteogenesis proximally and soft tissue distraction distally.

phalanx in favor of a mobile hallux. At 2 years' postoperation, the patient remains without symptoms and is active as a hospital-based physical therapist (**Fig. 3**).

CASE 2

Sometimes first ray complications present as just one component to a myriad of problems. Case 2 involves a 57-year-old prison inmate with chronic forefoot pain secondary to multilevel forefoot deformity as a result of multiple failed surgical interventions (**Fig. 4**).

In this case, consideration was given to transmetatarsal amputation. The patient, however, felt that an amputation could potentially make him more vulnerable to assault in his current environment as a federal prisoner. Therefore, an attempt at forefoot reconstruction was entertained. Presenting global deformities included a hallux malleus secondary to a malunion of the first metatarsophalangeal joint (MPJ) arthrodesis site, subluxed lesser MPJs, and hammertoe deformities. Correction entailed takedown of the first MPJ fusion site; arthrodesis of the hallus interphalangeal joint; resection of the second, third, and fifth metatarsal heads; and proximal interphalangeal joint arthrodesis of the lesser digits. The patient was doing well at 16 months post-op at which time he was lost to followup because of transfer to a minimum security facility (**Fig. 5**).

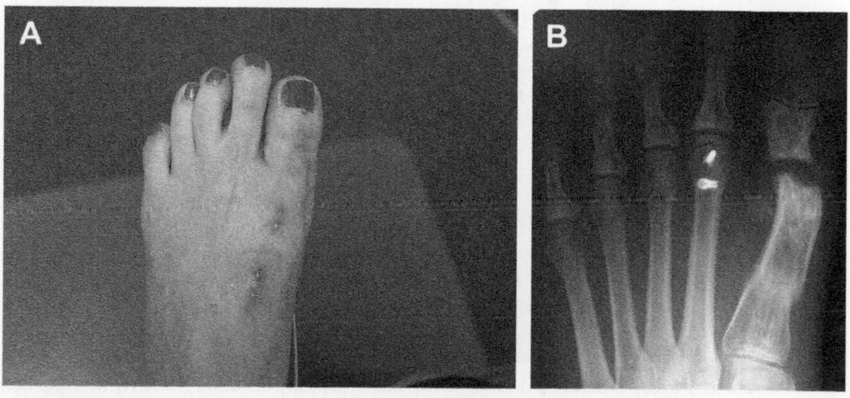

Fig. 3. (*A*) Final clinical appearance of case 1. (*B*) Note improved parabola.

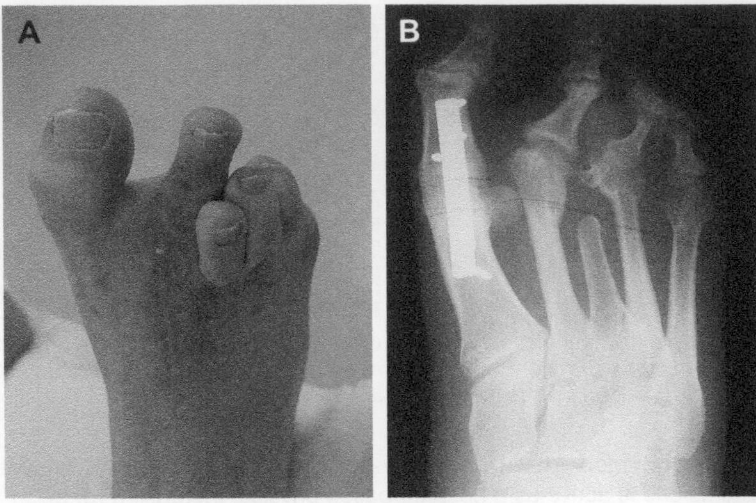

Fig. 4. Clinical (*A*) and radiographic (*B*) appearance from case 2 of a multilevel forefoot deformity as result of multiple surgical misadventures.

CASE 3

Case 3 involves a 62-year-old female homemaker who previously presented with a complaint of bunion pain and fourth digit hammertoe to an outside orthopedic clinic. The patient's index procedure included a first metatarsal head exostectomy with Akin osteotomy and a shortening procedure of the fourth metatarsal. Over the next 3 years, this created severe instability to the forefoot with resultant arthrosis deformans of the first MPJ, predislocation of the second MPJ, metatarsalgia, and hammertoe formation (**Fig. 6**).

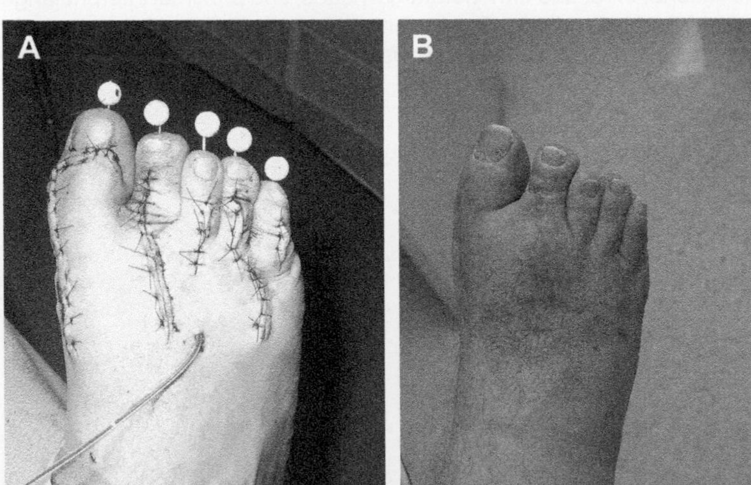

Fig. 5. Immediate postoperative (*A*) and long-term (*B*) appearance following aggressive forefoot reconstruction in case 2.

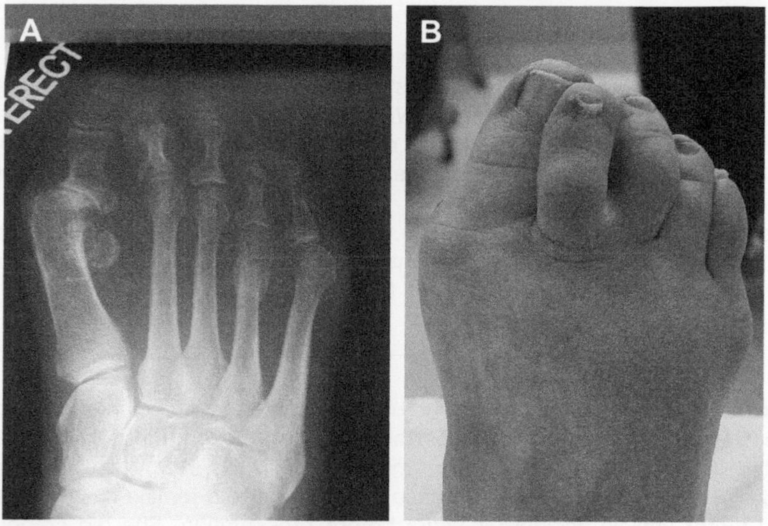

Fig. 6. Radiographic (*A*) and clinical (*B*) appearance of patient in case 3 after iatrogenic first MPJ arthrosis deformans and skewed metatarsal parabola.

Correction entailed extensive forefoot reconstruction via modified Austin osteotomy, hemi-implant arthroplasty, shortening osteotomies of the second and third rays, and hammertoe corrections via second and third proximal interphalangeal joint arthrodesis. The patient was doing well at 24-month follow-up (**Fig. 7**).

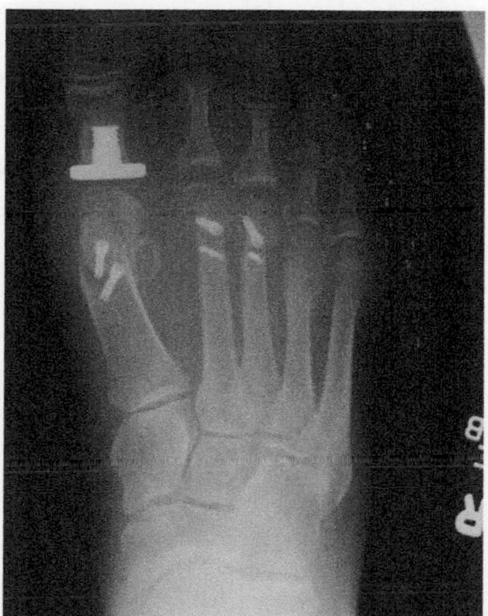

Fig. 7. Final correction in case 3 via modified Austin bunionectomy, hemi-implant arthroplasty, and metatarsal osteotomies.

CASE 4

Case 4 involves a 17-year-old female with juvenile hallux abductovalgus whose index procedure was a closing base wedge osteotomy and whose head procedure corrected for proximal articular set angle. Within 12 months of her original procedure, her hallux abductovalgus deformity had returned. Clearly her index deformity was the result of an atavistic and hypermobile first MCJ. Thus the index procedure was doomed from the start.

Correction entailed a modified Lapidus with interpositional allogenic bone graft to prevent excessive shortening. The patient was followed for 36 months and was released from our clinic without complaints (**Fig. 8**).

CASE 5

Lisfranc fracture dislocations are missed up to 20% of the time in the emergency department. Painful posttraumatic osteoarthritis is often the long-term sequel of these neglected injuries. When conservative measures fail, the only viable option is an arthrodesising type of procedure. In case 5, a 57-year-old female sustained a low-velocity motor vehicle accident 7 years before presentation. She did complain of midfoot pain at the initial presentation to the emergency department. Radiographs were ordered at the time and they were read as negative for fracture or dislocation. The initial treatment simply consisted of rest, ice, compression, and elevation for a short period followed by return to activity as tolerated. The patient began to experience new midfoot pain about 6 weeks after the index event. She was subsequently diagnosed with a neglected Lisfranc fracture/dislocation with new-onset osteoarthritis. She failed conservative treatment with orthotics and a series of local injections and oral nonsteroidal anti-inflammatory drugs. She then underwent an isolated midfoot arthrodesis. At 20 weeks' postoperation she continued to complain of pain to the midfoot. Clinically she had obvious transverse plane abduction deformity at the tarsometatarsal joint level. Subsequent CT revealed a nonunion across the affected joints. Radiographs reveal a transverse plane deformity with elevation of the first ray. The patient opted for revision-limited tarsometatarsal joint arthrodesis. The procedure was performed with two dorsal incisions, care being taken to keep the neurovascular

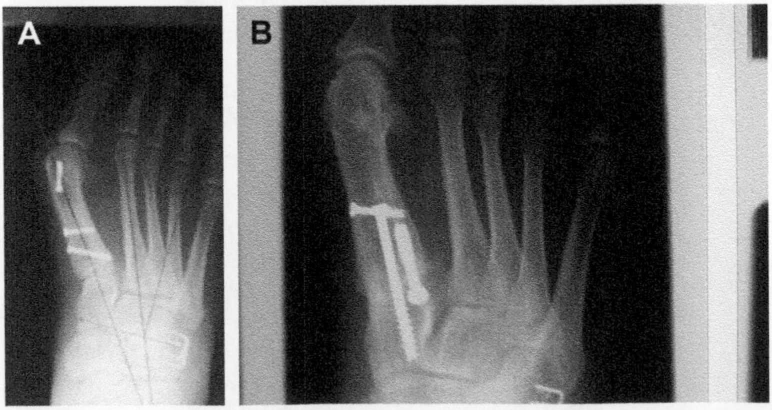

Fig. 8. Pre- (*A*) and postoperation (*B*) radiographs from case 4 of juvenile hallux abductovalgus deformity that quickly recurred as a result of poor procedure selection. Correction entailed Lapidus arthrodesis with distraction bone block graft.

bundle centered within the elevated fasiocutaneous bridge. Enhancement of the arthrodesis site was obtained via demineralized bone matrix and platelet gel concentrate. Fixation consisted of compression screw fixation and a dorsally placed locking plate designed for the unique anatomy of the medial midfoot. At 10 weeks' postoperation there was good fusion and the patient slowly returned to her activities of daily living (**Figs. 9–11**).

DISCUSSION

Complications of the first ray generally entail problems with alignment or length as an end result of infection, delayed union, nonunion, mal-union, avascular necrosis, poor choice of index reconstructive procedure, or loss of reduction following posttraumatic reconstruction. The authors have found that certain reproducible strategies exist to address each of these entities.

In the case of deep bone infection, initial aggressive treatment via debridement and culture-directed antibiosis is paramount. Resection of large infected bone segments can be stabilized with external fixation in combination with intercalary antibiotic bone cement or beads for 6 weeks of total therapy. Subsequent surgical intervention entails either bone grafting or proximal distraction osteogenesis.

In the case of nonunion, such as might be seen with Lapidus arthrodesis or closing base wedge osteotomy, the authors obtain a technetium bone scan to assess the potential for local biologic activity. If the scan is positive, then often an external bone stimulator along with non–weight bearing and immobilization will suffice. If the bone scan is "cold," then the best option may be to revise the nonunion site via debridement with bone grafting and appropriate fixation. Catagni[5] has also described the successful application of external fixation in the treatment of hypertrophic nonunions.

Complications of the first ray can be devastating to the patient from a functional standpoint. However, aggressive initial treatment followed by well thought out reconstructive strategies can often produce favorable results despite the severity of the index presentation.

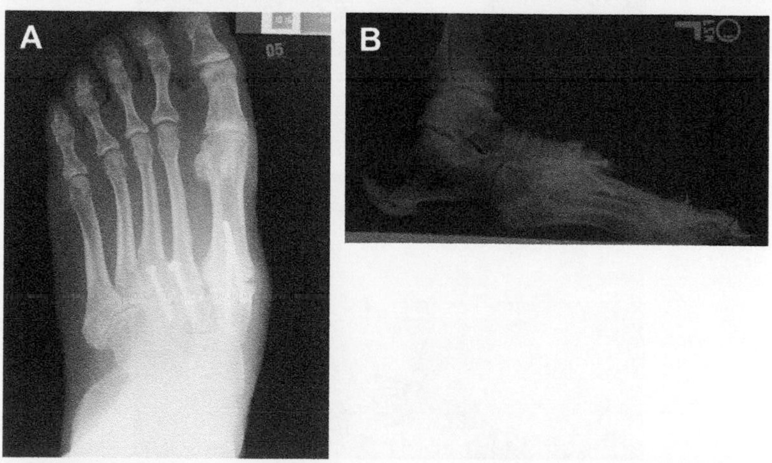

Fig. 9. (*A* and *B*) Radiographic images from case 5 of nonunion lesser tarsometatarsal joint following missed Lisfranc injury.

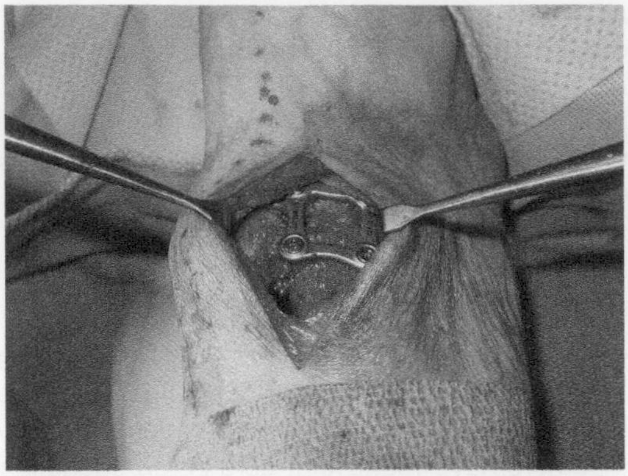

Fig. 10. Intraoperative image of dorsal tarsometatarsal joint fusion locking plate from case 5.

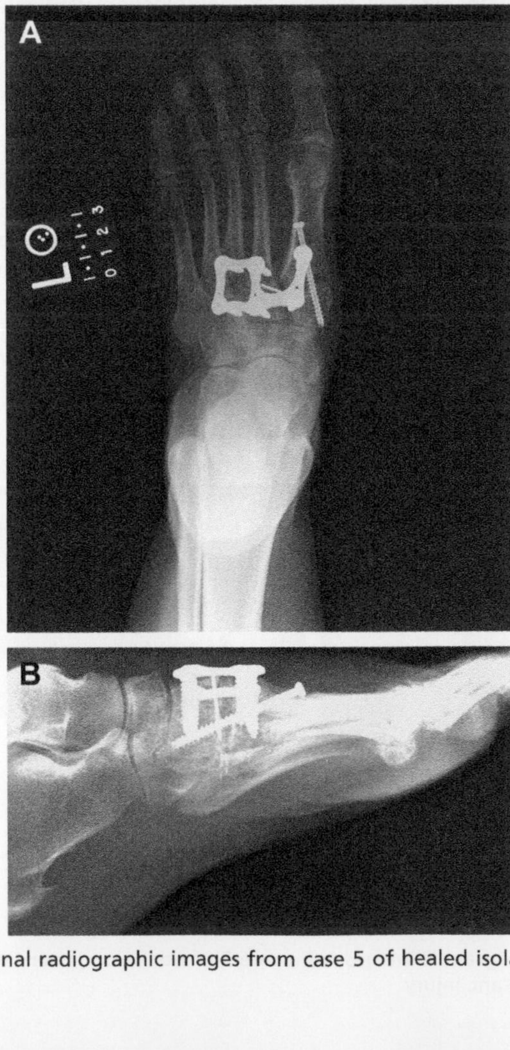

Fig. 11. (*A* and *B*) Final radiographic images from case 5 of healed isolated tarsometatarsal joint arthrodesis.

REFERENCES

1. Sammarco VJ, Acevedo J. Stability and fixation techniques in first metatarsal osteotomies. Foot Ankle Clin 2001;6(3):409–32.
2. Acevedo JI, Sammarco J, Boucher HR, et al. Mechanical comparison of cyclic loading in five different first metatarsal shaft osteotomies. Foot Ankle Int 2002; 23:711–6.
3. Austin DW, Leventen EO. A new osteotomy for hallux valgus: a horizontally directed V displacement osteotomy of the metatatarsal head for hallux valgus and primus varus. Clin Orthop 1981;157:25–30.
4. Lagaay PM, Hamilton GA, Ford LA, et al. Rates of revision surgery using chevron-Austin osteotomy, Lapidus arthrodesis, and closing base wedge osteotomy for correction of hallux valgus deformity. J Foot Ankle Surg 47(4):267–72, Epub 2008 May 9.
5. Catagni MA, Guerreschi F, Holman JA, et al. Distraction osteogenesis in the treatment of stiff hypertrophic nonunions using the Ilizarov apparatus. Clin Orthop Relat Res 1994 Apr;(301):159–63.

Revision of Failed Flatfoot Surgery

Michael S. Lee, DPM, FACFAS[a,b,*], Jared M. Maker, BS[a]

KEYWORDS

- Failed flatfoot • Flatfoot • Pes valgus
- Revision surgery • Recurrence

Revision of the malaligned flatfoot correction poses a significant challenge for the foot and ankle surgeon. The complex nature of the presenting deformity, the biomechanical consequences, and the relation between the osseous and soft tissue structures contribute to a deformity that often varies in degree of severity, nature, and location of pain and instability. The foot and ankle literature is replete with various techniques implemented to correct this triplane deformity.[1–5] The wide range of opinions and literature dedicated to this clinical entity demonstrates the complex nature of the human flatfoot and the techniques for deformity correction. There remains no accepted treatment algorithm or paradigm.[6] Addressing failed flatfoot surgery is made especially difficult because of the lack of uniform approaches to the primary deformity.

Primary correction of the adult acquired flatfoot is a well-studied and documented clinical condition; revisional flatfoot surgery, conversely, is a topic that has little scientific literature to support or guide the foot and ankle surgeon. Much of the literature deals with complications of flatfoot surgery, whereas little literature addresses revision of failed or malaligned flatfoot surgery.

This article attempts to break down various aspects of this deformity and each one's contribution to surgical failure, the role of procedure selection in flatfoot correction, and techniques used in revisional flatfoot surgery. Admittedly, some of the senior author's opinions are theoretic or dogmatic. More scientific work is clearly warranted in the area of revisional flatfoot surgery.

DEFORMITY CONSIDERATIONS

Ankle joint equinus has been shown to be present in up to 96% of all patients with biomechanically induced foot pain. It remains extremely underdiagnosed and is one of the most undertreated of all foot and ankle conditions.[7] The role of equinus with regard to the flatfoot deformity, adult and pediatric, has been continuously debated.

[a] College of Podiatric Medicine and Surgery, Des Moines University, Des Moines, IA, USA
[b] Central Iowa Orthopaedics, Foot and Ankle Surgeon, 1601 NW 114th Street, Suite 142, Des Moines, IA 50325, USA
* Corresponding author. Central Iowa Orthopaedics, Foot and Ankle Surgeon, 1601 NW 114th Street, Suite 142, Des Moines, IA 50325.
E-mail address: mlee.cio@mac.com (M.S. Lee).

Clin Podiatr Med Surg 26 (2009) 47–58
doi:10.1016/j.cpm.2008.09.002
podiatric.theclinics.com

Compensation for an ankle equinus typically results in subtalar and midtarsal joint pronation.[8] Thordarson and colleagues[9] demonstrated a threefold increase in the arch-deforming effect of the Achilles tendon over the arch-supporting effect of the posterior tibial tendon.

Failure to correct this soft tissue contracture may contribute to a residual deformity and is a common cause of undercorrected deformities. Hibbs[10] was the first to advocate a tendo–Achilles tendon lengthening procedure as part of the treatment for a pes planus deformity. With equinus, the Achilles tendon forces the calcaneus in a valgus position and limits subtalar joint inversion.[11] To position the calcaneus in a rectus position with any flatfoot reconstruction properly, a posterior muscle group lengthening procedure should be considered.

Degeneration of the posterior tibial tendon has been attributed to many hypotheses.[12–15] A zone of hypovascularity was identified 1.4 cm immediately distal to the tip of the medial malleolus.[14] This hypovascular zone was once thought to contribute to the degeneration of the posterior tibial tendon. A more recent study by Prado and colleagues[15] using a special staining technique demonstrated that the hypovascular zone does not exist. They believed that posterior tibial tendon failure was the result of mechanical stress rather than ischemia attributable to hypovascularity.

The spring ligament is a complex structure containing four components: the inferior calcaneonavicular ligament, the superomedial calcaneonavicular ligament, the anterior portion of the deltoid ligament, and the posterior tibial tendon.[16] This ligament complex forms an articular sling around the talar head. Its strength has been shown to be equivalent to the strength of the lateral collateral ligaments of the ankle.[16] The spring ligament provides static support of the talar head, resisting medial and plantar subluxation. Attenuation of the spring ligament complex may accentuate the flatfoot deformity, and consideration for repair is warranted.

An unlocked midtarsal joint during midstance allows the concentric contraction of the Achilles tendon to plantarflex the hindfoot on the forefoot. This places significant overload on the posterior tibial tendon and the spring ligament in addition to the long and short plantar ligaments and the plantar aponeurosis.[17] This process results in "lateral peritalar subluxation."[18,19] This peritalar subluxation results in midfoot abduction and forefoot supinatus. In long-standing deformities, the forefoot supinatus may become a fixed varus deformity. Failure to recognize such a fixed position may result in improper procedure selection and a residual deformity (**Fig. 1**). Failure to address

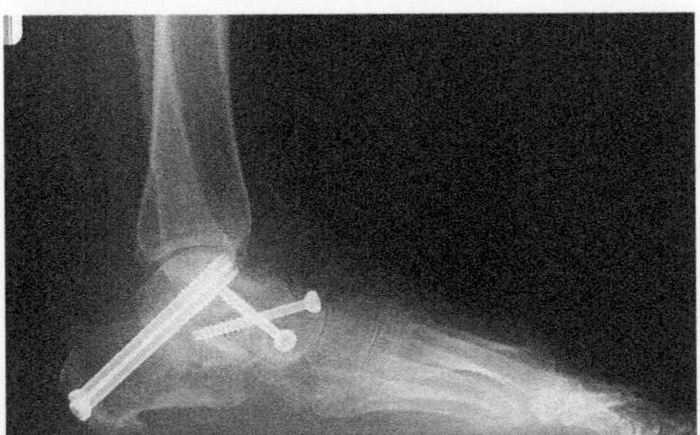

Fig.1. Double subtalar joint (STJ) and talonavicular joint (TNJ) arthrodesis of a severe flatfoot deformity demonstrates an undercorrected forefoot varus deformity with elevation of the first ray and lateral column overload.

a fixed forefoot varus may result in lateral column overload or even hallux rigidus attributable to an elevated first ray.

Faulting of the medial column in the adult acquired flatfoot may occur at the talonavicular joint, naviculocuneiform joint, or first metatarsocuneiform joint (MCJ).[20,21] The medial column has been described as a "post" for the talus.[21] With medial column faulting, the post is compromised, allowing increased peritalar subluxation.[20] In the authors' experience, the breach or faulting occurs at the naviculocuneiform joint in most adult acquired flatfoot cases. In some cases with concurrent hallux valgus deformity, the senior author has found the breach to occur more distally at the first MCJ. Failure to recognize and address the medial column faulting is a common problem, leading to undercorrection of the adult acquired flatfoot (**Fig. 2**).

Hindfoot valgus is well recognized in its role in the adult acquired flatfoot. The clinical and radiographic evaluation of hindfoot valgus in the adult acquired flatfoot has been well documented.[22,23] Realignment of the valgus hindfoot into a rectus position re-establishes the insertion of the Achilles tendon medial to the subtalar joint axis of motion, therefore increasing a supinatory action by the Achilles tendon. Additionally, a rectus heel exhibits less pronatory ground-reactive forces at heel strike.[24] Undercorrection of the hindfoot valgus limits these supinatory effects, whereas overcorrection can accentuate supination, leading to lateral column overload.

Ankle valgus signifies the final stage of the adult acquired flatfoot deformity.[25] Although infrequently encountered in most clinical practices, the foot and ankle surgeon must always be cognizant of this end-stage deformity. In cases demonstrating significant valgus malalignment, particularly nonreducible deformities, radiographs of the ankle should be obtained. Although the ankle may maintain adequate range of motion and lack clinical symptoms, a significant amount of valgus malalignment may be noted (**Fig. 3**). Failure to address the ankle valgus as part of the flatfoot reconstruction results in continued malalignment, calcaneal valgus, and progressive ankle arthrosis.

SURGICAL MALALIGNMENT

Surgical correction of the adult acquired flatfoot may fail for any number of reasons. With regard to malalignment, however, it has been the senior author's experience that a great number of these reconstructions fail because of four common errors. These include failure to recognize or adequately treat equinus, undercorrection of

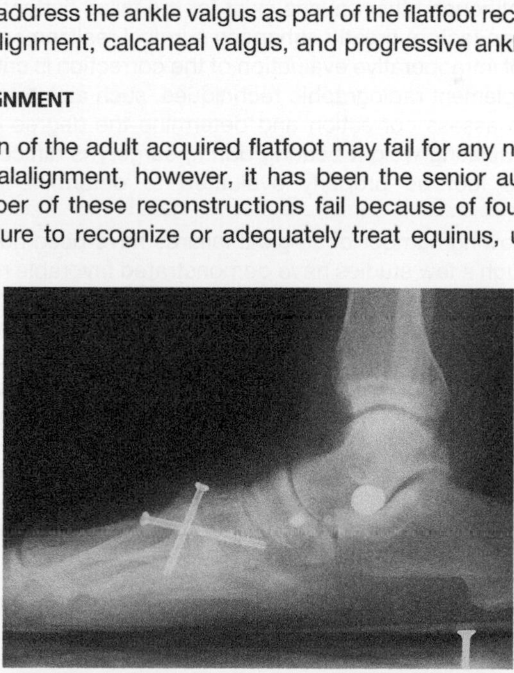

Fig. 2. Medial column faulting at the naviculocuneiform joint after flatfoot correction with MCJ arthrodesis, subtalar arthroereisis, and flexor digitorum longus (FDL) tendon transfer. Note the first ray elevation contributing to the medial column faulting.

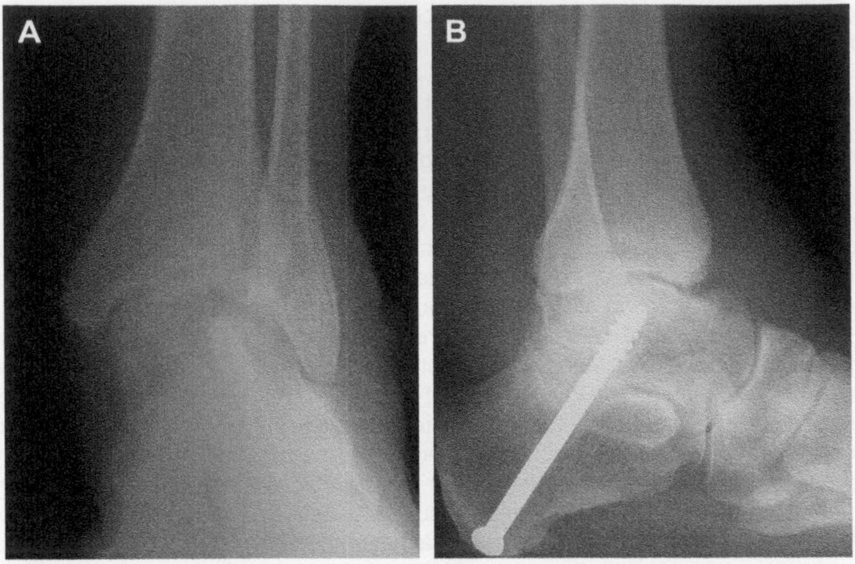

Fig. 3. (*A*) Valgus malalignment in a patient who recently underwent triple arthrodesis for a severe adult acquired flatfoot. (*B*) In the same patient, a lateral view demonstrates the triple arthrodesis with residual unrecognized ankle valgus malalignment.

the hindfoot valgus, failure to address the medial column faulting, or failure to recognize ankle valgus. Although other causes exist for the failed flatfoot correction, eliminating these common factors greatly enhances surgical realignment.

The importance of intraoperative evaluation of the correction is critical. The surgeon should routinely implement radiographic techniques, such as intraoperative hindfoot alignment views, to assess correction and determine the degree of residual deformity.[23] Although simulating weight bearing during surgery is difficult to achieve, it is imperative that the foot be properly evaluated to determine the adequacy of correction.

Additionally, a growing number of surgical failures have been noted after subtalar arthroereisis. Although a few studies have demonstrated favorable results with subtalar arthroereisis in the adult acquired flatfoot, more research is clearly warranted.[26–28] The procedure has limitations and is primarily indicated to correct hindfoot valgus by limiting subtalar joint eversion (**Fig. 4**).[29] Overuse of these implants has been noted because surgeons implement arthroereisis for all deformities rather than limiting its indications. The ease with which these implants are implanted and explanted may contribute to the recent increase in use. Limiting the use of these implants to the correction of frontal plane malalignment can limit complications and residual deformities.

REVISION CONSIDERATIONS

Paramount to addressing the residual flatfoot deformity is understanding exactly what procedures were implemented during the index procedure. It is not enough to rely on the patient's history. A great deal of information may be gleaned from the clinical and radiographic examination, including incision placement, previous osteotomies and fixation, and deformity alignment. The foot and ankle surgeon should make every attempt to procure the original operative report. The operative report may shed

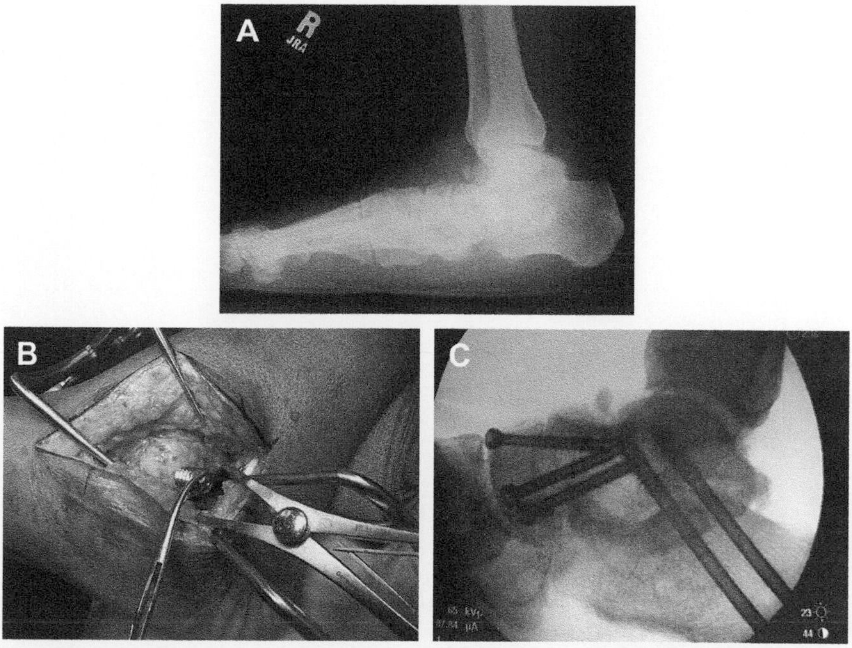

Fig. 4. (*A*) Male patient who weighed 305 lb and had a recurrent flatfoot after subtalar arthroereisis and flexor transfer. (*B*) Medial approach to the subtalar joint with removal of the subtalar implant. (*C*) Medial approach subtalar and talonavicular joint arthrodesis.

particularly useful information regarding the types of tendon lengthening or repair techniques and the potential contribution to the residual deformity.

Equinus should be carefully evaluated. It has been the senior author's experience that in a great number of failed (undercorrected) flatfoot operations, a common thread has been inadequate or absence of equinus correction during the index surgery. Therefore, it is particularly important that the role of equinus be fully evaluated and addressed with the residual flatfoot deformity. In most cases of revisional flatfoot surgery, a gastrocnemius recession is implemented for equinus correction by the senior author. In cases in which a tendo–Achilles tendon lengthening may have been attempted with inadequate correction, the scar tissue in the Achilles tendon makes proper lengthening (especially with a percutaneous approach) difficult. Moving more proximally into the gastrocnemius aponeurosis provides adequate correction, often through virgin tissues with limited morbidity.[30,31] Most often, a medial approach to the gastrocnemius aponeurosis, as previously described, is used (**Fig. 5**).[32]

Isolated flexor tendon transfer has been shown to provide symptomatic relief, but residual osseous deformity typically leads to a recurrence of deformity and symptoms.[33] A flexor digitorum longus (FDL) tendon transfer does not balance the opposing forces of the peroneus brevis tendon entirely, causing various researchers to recommend the addition of a calcaneal osteotomy.[3,4,24] The failure of the tendon transfer may be attributable to the ligamentous attenuation. Additionally, if the forefoot varus is not recognized, the tendon transfer may fail because the medial post is insufficient to prevent subtalar joint eversion.[33]

In cases of residual or recurrent flatfoot in which symptoms persist along the course of the posterior tibial tendon or spring ligament, revisional flexor transfer may be

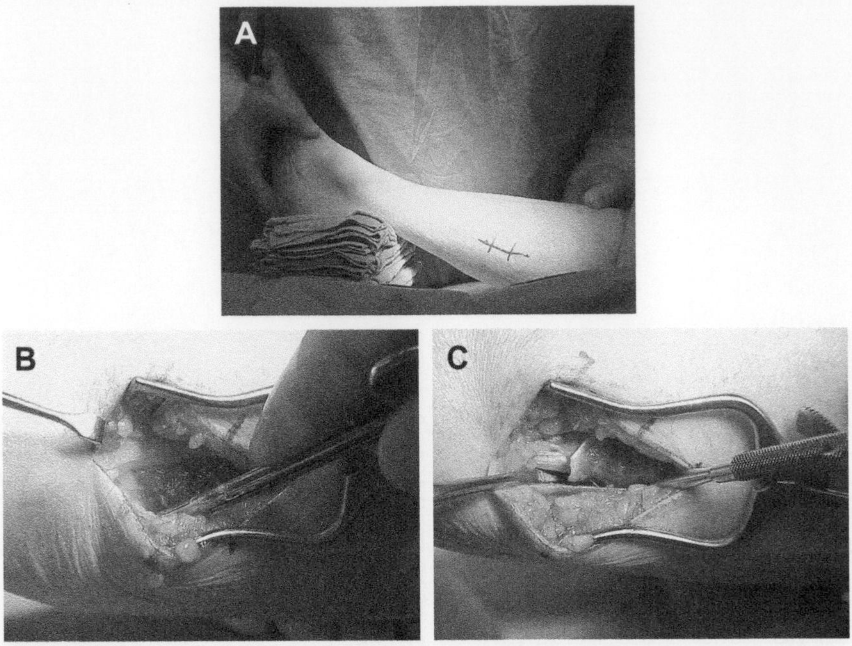

Fig. 5. (*A*) Medial incision for a gastrocnemius recession. (*B*) Visualization of the gastrocnemius myotendinous junction. (*C*) Medial-to-lateral transection of the gastrocnemius aponeurosis. (*From* Lee MS. Medial approach to the severe valgus foot. Clin Podiatr Med Surg 2007;24:736–7; with permission.)

considered. In most cases, however, the persistent symptoms occur laterally, typically in the sinus tarsi region or by causing subfibular impingement pain. In these cases, the surgeon must carefully determine whether a flexor tendon transfer remains a viable option. Procedure selection may also play a critical role in determining whether a flexor transfer is warranted. When a triple, double, or talonavicular fusion is selected for revisional surgery, transfer of the FDL tendon results in no biomechanical advantage or improvement.

In cases of residual hindfoot valgus, particularly in cases that maintain adequate or supple subtalar joint range of motion, calcaneal osteotomies may be beneficial. Undercorrection of the posterior calcaneal displacement osteotomy (PCDO) with less than 10 mm of posterior tuber translation has been shown to lead to subjective and objectively poorer results (**Fig. 6**).[24] Revising such an osteotomy with more appropriate alignment and correction is relatively simple to achieve. More often, however, the Evans calcaneal osteotomy may be used to correct the residual hindfoot valgus deformity with a supple subtalar joint range of motion. The Evans osteotomy provides more significant forefoot abduction and forefoot varus correction than the PCDO, and is therefore more dynamic in its correction of the residual flatfoot deformity.[22,34–36]

Many patients who have residual flatfeet present not only with a continued hindfoot valgus but with collapse of the medial column or a naviculocuneiform breach or sag. This often represents compensation for the forefoot varus deformity.[11] The medial column has been somewhat overlooked with regard to its role in the flatfoot deformity. Most medial column procedures have traditionally been viewed as "adjunctive" or "ancillary" to calcaneal osteotomies. In many cases, failure to correct the medial

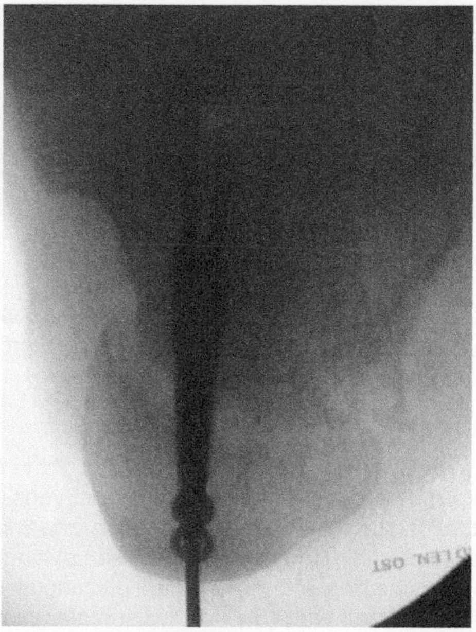

Fig. 6. Undercorrection of a PCDO with less than 10 mm of medial realignment noted on the axial view.

column faulting has led to a biomechanically unstable foot, resulting in residual deformity. Evaluation of the medial column and correction of any instability therein plays a significant role in correcting the residual flatfoot.[20] The naviculocuneiform joint (NCJ) fusion may provide significant correction in the transverse and sagittal planes. Joint preparation with curettage allows one to activate the windlass mechanism to plantarflex and adduct the forefoot on the hindfoot, correcting residual deformity (**Fig. 7**).[20]

Medial column sag in some cases of residual flatfoot may present more distal in the MCJ. In cases of concurrent hallux valgus, this is particularly true. In such cases, MCJ arthrodesis with sagittal and transverse plane correction may be warranted (**Fig. 8**).

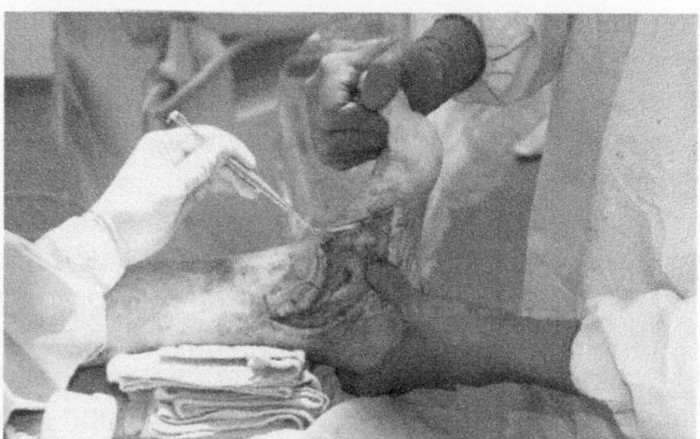

Fig. 7. Activation of the windlass mechanism for reduction of the deformity and temporary pinning. Pressure is placed on the navicular tuberosity with the left thumb to assist in correction. (*From* Budny AM, Grossman JP. Naviculocuneiform arthrodesis. Clin Podiatr Med Surg 2007;24:759; with permission.)

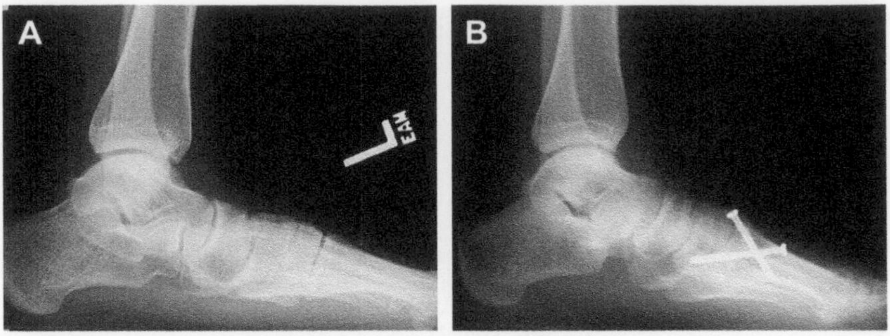

Fig. 8. (*A*) Preoperative flatfoot with concurrent hallux valgus. (*B*) Postoperative lateral radiograph with Evans calcaneal osteotomy and first MCJ fusion.

Care should be taken to limit joint resection from the base of the first metatarsal when a first metatarsocuneiform arthrodesis is coupled with an Evans calcaneal osteotomy so as not to weaken the insertion and strength of the peroneal longus tendon.

In cases of previous isolated hindfoot fusion with residual hindfoot valgus, a PCDO is more often used to bring the posterior tuber of the calcaneus in more neutral alignment. Wedging of the subtalar joint after an isolated subtalar joint arthrodesis may be considered, but in cases of residual valgus, this requires a laterally based opening wedge with graft or a medially based closing wedge. Revisional wedging through a fused subtalar joint is more likely to be considered in cases of varus malalignment or overcorrection of the adult flatfoot.

Lateral column lengthening by an Evans osteotomy or calcaneocuboid joint distraction arthrodesis can result in lateral column pain. This is particularly true if the forefoot varus is not corrected. Ideally, lengthening of the lateral column forces the peroneus longus tendon, long plantar ligament, and plantar fascia to restore the arch and correct forefoot varus. Some researchers have advocated using a smaller trapezoid-shaped graft for the Evans osteotomy to plantarflex and adduct the midfoot and forefoot.[37] If the forefoot remains in varus, consideration of a medial column fusion is warranted.

An isolated talonavicular joint arthrodesis is particularly difficult to manage. Undercorrection and overcorrection of the adult acquired flatfoot are difficult to manage once the talonavicular joint is fused in malalignment. Almost all procedures correct the flatfoot by rotating the hindfoot (calcaneus) or the forefoot or midfoot (navicular) around the talus. Therefore, if the talonavicular joint has been arthrodesed, any further reconstruction is limited because the foot cannot be allowed to rotate around the talonavicular joint. In cases of malunion of the talonavicular joint, a takedown osteotomy may be completed (**Fig. 9**).

The long-term results of triple arthrodesis were evaluated by Graves and colleagues;[38] all deformities involved nonneuromuscular conditions, including posterior tibial tendon dysfunction and rheumatoid arthritis. Eighty-two percent of patients expressed satisfaction with the procedure, but 41% expressed no improvement in the distance they could walk after surgery. Patient acceptance of triple arthrodesis, even in cases with appropriate correction, has been less than predictable.[38–40] The loss of frontal plane motion through the subtalar joint presents significant problems for the patient clinically, especially on uneven ground. Valgus or varus malalignment after triple arthrodesis can present difficulties even while standing.[41] Long term, especially in patients with malalignment, the development of arthrosis in the ankle or midtarsal joints may become problematic.[42]

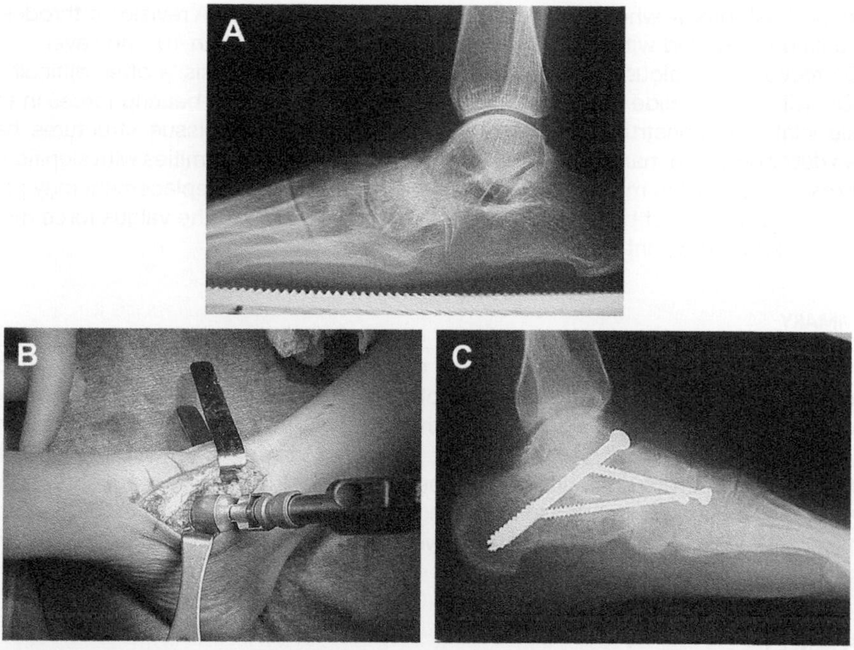

Fig. 9. (*A*) Twenty-year-old woman after talonavicular arthrodesis and no posterior muscle group lengthening with residual undercorrected flatfoot. (*B*) Takedown osteotomy of the talonavicular joint. (*C*) Realignment and triple arthrodesis after surgery.

Revision of the failed triple arthrodesis presents a difficult challenge.[11] Haddad and colleagues[42] have previously presented an algorithm to fix the residual deformity after a triple arthrodesis systematically. The algorithm focuses on the fixed residual deformity, working from the hindfoot to the forefoot. Particular attention is paid to the residual hindfoot varus or valgus malalignment and to the amount of residual forefoot supinatus or varus.[42]

In cases of residual hindfoot valgus, Haddad and colleagues[42] advocate a PCDO. In cases of an overcorrected triple arthrodesis with calcaneal varus, however, a laterally based closing wedge with lateral translation of the posterior tuber of the calcaneus is recommended.[42] Intraoperative hindfoot alignment views should be used to confirm proper alignment and correction of the deformity.[23]

The midfoot malalignment can present significant problems if not properly addressed after realigning the hindfoot. A wedging osteotomy through the midtarsal joint has been advocated.[42] The senior author has found that patients have a residual naviculocuneiform fault in many cases, however, and addressing the residual deformity through this joint often leads to adequate correction without taking down a consolidated fusion site.

Rush[43] also addresses issues dealing with failed flatfoot surgery. With hindfoot procedures, undercorrecting a hindfoot valgus is the primary cause for revision surgery. Valgus malalignment with a subtalar fusion or triple arthrodesis leads to failure of the deltoid ligament and ankle degeneration. Realigning the hindfoot re-establishes medial stability and lessens the deteriorating forces applied to the deltoid ligament and posterior tibial tendon. Overcorrection of the hindfoot can cause a varus malalignment. Residual valgus or varus malalignment can be corrected with a posterior calcaneal osteotomy when the degree of malalignment is small. A revision arthrodesis is commonly needed with a residual hindfoot valgus greater than 10°, however.

Correction of a valgus ankle deformity after a triple arthrodesis is often difficult. A PCDO with medial slide may improve the distribution of weight-bearing forces in the ankle joint.[44] Reconstruction of the deltoid and medial soft tissue structures has been described.[43] In many cases, especially long-standing deformities with significant arthrosis, ankle fusion may be the only option. Total ankle joint replacement may provide more options, but balancing of the foot and elimination of the valgus force must be achieved before joint replacement.

SUMMARY

Revision of failed flatfoot surgery requires particular attention to detail. The surgeon must fully understand the presenting complaints of the patient, why the index procedure failed, and the ramifications of another surgical procedure. Goals of revising failed flatfoot surgery focus on achieving a plantigrade foot and imparting stability to the hindfoot and ankle. Little literature supports the foot and ankle surgeon in his or her decision-making process, complicating revision surgery further. In general, the surgeon should perform the least invasive procedure while decreasing pain and improving function.

REFERENCES

1. Coetzee JC, Castro MD. The indications and biomechanical rationale for various hindfoot procedures in the treatment of posterior tibialis tendon dysfunction. Foot Ankle Clin 2003;8:453–9.
2. Harper MC. Talonavicular arthrodesis for the acquired flatfoot in the adult. Clin Orthop Relat Res 1999;365:65–8.
3. Myerson MS, Corrigan J, Thompson F, et al. Tendon transfer combined with calcaneal osteotomy for treatment of posterior tibial tendon insufficiency: a radiological investigation. Foot Ankle Int 1995;16:712–8.
4. Mosier-LaClair S, Pomeroy G, Manoli A. Operative treatment of the difficult stage 2 adult acquired flatfoot deformity. Foot Ankle Clin 2001;6:95–119.
5. Weinraub GM, Heilala MA. Adult flatfoot/posterior tibial tendon dysfunction: outcomes analysis of surgical treatment utilizing an algorithmic approach. J Foot Ankle Surg 2000;39:359–64.
6. Hiller L, Pinney S. Surgical treatment of acquired flatfoot deformity: what is the state of practice among academic foot and ankle surgeons in 2002. Foot Ankle Int 2003;24:701–5.
7. Hill RS. Ankle equinus: prevalence and linkage to common foot pathology. J Am Podiatr Med Assoc 1995;85:295–300.
8. Meszaros A, Caudell G. The surgical management of equinus in the adult acquired flatfoot. Clin Podiatr Med Surg 2007;24:667–85.
9. Thordarson DB, Schmotzer H, Chon J, et al. Dynamic support of the human longitudinal arch. A biomechanical evaluation. Clin Orthop Relat Res 1995;316:165–72.
10. Hibbs RA. Muscle bound feet. New York Medical Journal 1914;17C:797–9.
11. Toolan BC. The treatment of failed reconstruction for adult acquired flat foot deformity. Foot Ankle Clin 2003;8(3):647–54.
12. Petersen W, Hohmann G, Stein V, et al. The blood supply of the posterior tibial tendon. J Bone Joint Surg Br 2002;84:141–4.

13. Uchimaya E, Kitaoka HB, Fujii T, et al. Gliding resistance of the posterior tibial tendon. Foot Ankle Int 2006;27:723–6.
14. Frey C, Shereff M, Greenidge N. Vascularity of the posterior tibial tendon. J Bone Joint Surg Am 1990;72:884–8.
15. Prado MP, Carvalho AE, Rodriques CJ, et al. Vascular density of the posterior tibial tendon: a cadaver study. Foot Ankle Int 2006;27:628–31.
16. Davis WH, Sobel M, Ci Carlo EF, et al. Gross, histological, and microvascular anatomy and biomechanical testing of the spring ligament complex. Foot Ankle Int 1996;17:95–102.
17. Richie DH. Biomechanics and clinical analysis of the adult acquired flatfoot. Clin Podiatr Med Surg 2007;24:617–44.
18. Hansen ST. Progressive symptomatic flat foot (lateral peritalar subluxation). In: Hansen ST, editor. Functional reconstruction of the foot and ankle. Philadelphia: Lippincott Williams & Wilkins; 2000. p. 195–207.
19. Van Boerum DH, Sangeorzan BJ. Biomechanics and pathophysiology of flat foot. Foot Ankle Clin 2003;8:419–30.
20. Budny AM, Grossman JP. Naviculocuneiform arthrodesis. Clin Podiatr Med Surg 2007;24:753–63.
21. Greisberg J, Assal M, Hansen S, et al. Isolated medial column stabilization improves alignment in adult acquired flatfoot. Clin Orthop Relat Res 2005;435: 197–202.
22. Lee MS, Vanore JV, Thomas JL, et al. Clinical practice guideline adult flatfoot panel. Diagnosis and treatment of adult flatfoot. J Foot Ankle Surg 2005;44: 78–113.
23. Catanzariti AR, Mendicino RW, Whitaker JM, et al. Realignment considerations in the triple arthrodesis. J Am Podiatr Med Assoc 2005;95:13–7.
24. Catanzariti AR, Lee MS, Mendicino RW. Posterior calcaneal displacement osteotomy for adult acquired flatfoot deformities. J Foot Ankle Surg 2000;9:2–9.
25. Myerson M. Adult acquired flatfoot deformity: treatment of dysfunction of the posterior tibial tendon. J Bone Joint Surg 1996;78(A):780–802.
26. Viladot R, Pons M, Alvarez F, et al. Subtalar arthroereisis for posterior tibial tendon dysfunction: a preliminary report. Foot Ankle Int 2003;24:600–6.
27. Maxwell JR, Carro A, Sun C. Use of the Maxwell-Brancheau arthroereisis implant for the correction of posterior tibial tendon dysfunction. Clin Podiatr Med Surg 1999;16:479–89.
28. Needleman RL. A surgical approach for flexible flatfeet in adults including a subtalar arthroereisis with the MBA sinus tarsi implant. Foot Ankle Int 2006; 27:9–18.
29. Chang TJ, Lee J. Subtalar joint arthroereisis in adult-acquired flatfoot and posterior tibial tendon dysfunction. Clin Podiatr Med Surg 2007;24:687–97.
30. Sammarco GJ, Bagwe MR, Sammarco VJ, et al. The effects of unilateral gastrocsoleus recession. Foot Ankle Int 2006;27:508–11.
31. Rush SM, Ford LA, Hamilton GA. Morbidity associated with high gastrocnemius recession: retrospective review of 126 cases. J Foot Ankle Surg 2006;45:156–60.
32. Lee MS. Medial approach to the severe valgus foot. Clin Podiatr Med Surg 2007; 24:735–44.
33. Mann RA. Posterior tibial tendon dysfunction. Treatment by flexor digitorum longus transfer. Foot Ankle Clin 2001;6:77–87.
34. Evans D. Calcaneo-valgus deformity. J Bone Joint Surg Br 1975;57:270–8.
35. Phillips GE. A review of elongation of os calcis for flat feet. J Bone Joint Surg Br 1983;65:15–8.

36. Dollard MD, Marcinko DE, Lazerson A, et al. The Evans calcaneal osteotomy for correction of flexible flatfoot syndrome. J Foot Surg 1984;23:291–301.
37. Neufeld SK, Myerson MS. Complications of surgical treatments for adult flatfoot deformities. Foot Ankle Clin 2001;6:179–91.
38. Graves SC, Mann RA, Graves KO. Triple arthrodesis in older adults. Results after long-term follow-up care. J Bone Joint Surg Am 1993;75:355–62.
39. Mann RA, Van Manen JW, Wapner K, et al. Ankle fusion. Clin Orthop Relat Res 1991;268:49–55.
40. Sangeorzen BJ, Smith D, Veith R, et al. Triple arthrodesis using internal fixation in treatment of adult foot disorders. Clin Orthop 1993;294:299–307.
41. Haddad SL. Revision arthrodesis of the ankle and hindfoot. Foot Ankle Clin 1998; 3:51–70.
42. Haddad SL, Myerson MS, Pell RF, et al. Clinical and radiographic outcome of revision surgery for failed triple arthrodesis. Foot Ankle Int 1997;18:489–99.
43. Rush SM. Reconstructive options for failed flatfoot surgery. Clin Podiatr Med Surg 2007;24:779–88.
44. Jahss MH. Spontaneous rupture of the tibialis posterior tendon: clinical findings, tenographic studies, and a new technique of repair. Foot Ankle Int 1982;3: 158–64.

Revisional Hindfoot Arthrodesis

Lara J. Murphy, DPM, Robert W. Mendicino, DPM, FACFAS*, Alan R. Catanzariti, DPM, FACFAS

KEYWORDS

- Hindfoot arthrodesis • Revisional • Nonunion • Malunion

Since the late 1800s the hindfoot arthrodesis has been documented in literature for the treatment of painful arthritis, pes planovalgus, neuromuscular diseases, congenital and structural deformities, end-stage talar osteonecrosis, failed total ankle replacement, rheumatoid arthritis, and Charcot arthropathy.[1–15] Techniques have been described for the primary arthrodesis of a single joint to a complete pantalar fusion with early documented fusion rates being suboptimal.[2,16] With advancements in technology and fixation, however, current successful fusion rates range from 65% to 98%.[1,2,4–6,9,10,16–24] Complication rates have been described as high as 60% ranging from superficial wound infections to limb loss.[2,7,8,10,20,24,25] Nonunion and malunion of fusion sites are two of the most common and challenging of the complications. Hindfoot arthrodeses resulting from posttraumatic causes have been shown to have the most significant risk for nonunion.[26] Rates of nonunion vary with procedure, technique, and specific joint involved. Michelson and Curl published an extensive literature review that demonstrated the talonavicular joint as having the highest nonunion rate within a triple arthrodesis.[27,28] The ankle fusion portion of an attempted tibiotalocalcaneal arthrodesis has been shown to have the highest nonunion rate of the overall procedure.[8,9] Many authors have documented these specific complications but without commenting or recommending a resolution. This article provides a systematic approach to revisional hindfoot arthrodeses, focusing on patient evaluation, surgical technique, and postoperative treatment.

REASONS FOR FAILURE

On initial assessment, one should begin by performing an extensive review of the patient and surgical techniques performed as the possible causes of failure of the primary hindfoot arthrodesis. Most causes are multifactorial and not easily discernible, thus making it difficult to identify an origin of failure.

Department of Foot and Ankle Surgery, The Western Pennsylvania Hospital, 4800 Friendship Avenue North Tower First Floor, Pittsburgh, PA 15224, USA
* Corresponding author.
E-mail address: rmendicino@faiwp.com (R. Mendicino).

Clin Podiatr Med Surg 26 (2009) 59–78
doi:10.1016/j.cpm.2008.09.009
podiatric.theclinics.com

Fixation

Various fixation techniques have been described in the literature for hindfoot arthrodesis. Internal fixation, including plates, screws, intramedullary nails, and staples, have been used along with various forms of external fixation.[2,4–7,9,10,17–25,29–37] The extent and placement of fixation play significant roles in the stability and alignment of the arthrodesis site. Bennett and colleagues[8] in 2005 evaluated four methods of fixation for a tibiotalocalcaneal fusion. Using liquid metal strain gauges, they concluded that three crossed cancellous screws provided the greatest stability. A locked intramedullary nail with supplemental staple fixation was second. Previous to this, Berend and colleagues[38] in 1997 had concluded that an intramedullary nail had a significantly stiffer construct as compared with a double-crossed lag screw construct. Pelton and colleagues in 2006 evaluated the results of a tibiotalocalcaneal arthrodesis with the use of a dynamic retrograde intramedullary nail for fixation. They noted on follow-up evaluation a trend toward a higher nonunion rate in patients who had an increased nail-tibial angle.[5] Other forms of fixation, including inlay grafting, bone graft dowel arthrodesis, extra-articular arthrodesis, intramedullary fibular graft arthrodesis, and modified Blair arthrodesis, may be considered when evaluating an arthrodesis site.[23,39–43]

Surgical Approach

A traditional open approach is the most commonly performed technique; however, arthroscopic techniques have recently been described in the literature for hindfoot arthrodesis.[5,11,33,41,44–46] Both procedures provide comparative fusion rates for the ankle and subtalar joints; however, the arthroscopic approach can lend itself to decreased tissue manipulation, dissection, and operative time if performed with proper technique.[1,16,40,41] Arthroscopy has its limitations, with success limited to individuals who have minimal angular deformities. Collman and colleagues[16] in 2006 proposed that the two nonunions in their study may have occurred because of pre-existing ankle deformities.

Other considerations, including previous arthrodeses, must be taken into account. There has been a documented positive correlation between delayed unions and nonunions with previous adjacent sites of fusion.[6,31] Rosenfeld and colleagues presented a case of 4 nonunions within 100 cases of triple arthrodeses. Two of the 4 patients who had a subtalar nonunion had previously undergone an ipsilateral ankle fusion.[31]

Patient Selection

The patient's social and medical history can also have an influence on nonunion rates. Perlman and Thordarson[26] in 1999 noted a trend in ankle nonunions in patients who used tobacco, consumed alcohol, had a psychiatric disorder, or used illegal drugs. Ishikawa and colleagues[47] in 2002 documented a 2.7 times greater risk for developing a nonunion in patients who smoked compared with nonsmokers. Systemic diseases, including diabetes and rheumatoid arthritis, can also affect outcomes if not managed appropriately and patient compliance should also be taken into consideration because early weightbearing can lead to failure.[2,26,48]

Patient History

The patient's lifestyle, smoking history, nutritional status, and concomitant diseases all factor into the success of a surgical procedure. Research on the negative effects of tobacco on tissue and bone healing have been documented thoroughly in literature.[22,47,49] It is still uncertain, however, what length of time is needed between the cessation of tobacco and the operative procedure for the greatest effect.[47] At the author's institution, a protocol of 3 months' cessation of tobacco, including negative conitine and nicotine levels in the blood, is required before surgical intervention of a failed arthrodesis is considered.

The nutritional status of the patient should also be taken into consideration. Jensen and colleagues[50] in 1982 demonstrated a significant correlation between malnutrition and the development of complications postoperatively. They specifically focused on infection as the primary complication. They believed that a surgical procedure should be delayed until a more thorough nutritional work-up could be obtained if the patient had undergone a previous surgical procedure within 6 months, had a serum albumin of less than 3.4 gm/dL, or had a total lymphocyte count of less than 1500 cells/μL. Further blood work and a nutrition consult may be needed to add supplemental nutrition for an optimal healing environment.

Diabetes mellitus and rheumatoid arthritis are two major systemic diseases a patient may present with on evaluation. For a successful outcome it is imperative that blood glucose levels are tightly monitored. Medications, including immunosuppressants for rheumatoid arthritis, must be scrutinized carefully before surgical intervention. Many times these can increase wound dehiscence and infection rate if continued. Discussions with the primary care physician about the necessary dosages required should take place preoperatively. Bone stock in this patient population is usually poor and must be considered when choosing fixation. With any foot and ankle procedure, a multidisciplinary approach should be taken and all medical professionals participating in the care of your patient should be contacted and provide medical clearance for the patient before any extensive reconstruction.

PHYSICAL EXAMINATION

Because of the revisional nature of all procedures one must thoroughly evaluate not only the osseous structures but also the soft tissues involved. This evaluation may dictate choice of procedure, incision placement, and type of fixation. Noninvasive vascular studies, including pulse volume recordings, should be ordered if there is any question in vascularity. Many times the primary procedure was performed by a previous surgeon and therefore soft tissue structures that may have been traumatized or released are unknown. Any open lesions or draining sinuses must be examined and cultured. Further testing, including WBC-labeled bone scans or MR, should be ordered if needed to evaluate the extent of the infectious process. Symptoms relating to chronic regional pain syndrome may require assessment by a pain specialist before any surgical intervention.

Patients should be evaluated standing and during ambulation. Proximal joints, including the ankle and knee, should be assessed for any malalignment. Any component of equinus should be corrected at the time of surgical procedure. Manual muscle testing and range of motion of adjacent joints should be assessed. An ankle fusion requires adequate compensatory subtalar joint motion and a rearfoot arthrodesis relies on the midtarsal complex. Our own previous studies have found that patients who have limited preoperative motion at adjacent joints to the arthrodesis site demonstrated a greater likelihood for poor postoperative function. In a patient who has malalignment the compensatory motion may have been exaggerated and result in early degeneration.[51] Diagnostic local blocks are routinely given at the authors' institution to evaluate the level of the joint involvement and radiographs are used to evaluate quantitative angular measures to assess for malalignment.[51]

The patient should also be evaluated by physical therapy before any surgical intervention for the ability to remain nonweightbearing for the postoperative period. This assessment may help with the decision for possible postoperative placement in a subacute care or rehabilitation facility.

The foot and ankle are best evaluated with CT, MR, and plain radiographic imaging. A CT scan is used for evaluation of bony incorporation across the previous fusion site. An MRI can evaluate for any avascular necrosis, osteomyelitis, and if the nonunion demonstrates any hypertrophic or atrophic characteristics. Easley and colleagues[22] in 2000 discovered a positive correlation between the extent of avascular bone and union rate of the subtalar joint. If there was greater than 2 mm of avascular subchondral bone at the fusion site then there was an increased risk for nonunion. This risk was especially significant in revisional cases and sites with posttraumatic causes.

Specialized long leg calcaneal axial and hindfoot alignment sagittal plane views and standard radiographs should be obtained for evaluation of a malunion and nonunion. The long leg calcaneal axial view displays the relationship between the leg and the calcaneus and provides a clear view of the subtalar joint. The hindfoot alignment view provides visualization of the ankle joint allowing evaluation for any malalignment between the tibia and ankle.[51–56] These examinations can also be performed in the operating room (OR). Other specialty radiographs can be considered, including Johnson and colleagues'[57] hindfoot alignment view and the Coleman block test to evaluate for any forefoot deformity. If available erect lower limb radiographs of the full lower body are also recommended to evaluate for the center of rotation of angulation (CORA) in malaligned arthrodeses and rule out the possibility of any proximal malalignment or deformity.[56]

On evaluation of the lateral ankle view, the mid-diaphyseal line of the tibia should coincide with the lateral process of the talus. Other angles that should be evaluated include the plantigrade angle, the calcaneal inclination angle, the talar declination angle, the talocalcaneal angle, and the talo–first metatarsal angle.[53]

The anteroposterior view of the foot should include the talo–first metatarsal angle and the talocalcaneal angle for evaluation of any transverse deformity.[53]

With a thorough radiographic evaluation, the level of the deformity can be determined and necessary information provided for surgical planning. Overall bone quality and adjacent joint disease can also be assessed.

PATIENT AND SURGEON EXPECTATIONS AND GOALS

Before any surgical intervention the goals and expectations of each participant need to be expressed. The primary goal for any revisional surgery is to provide the patient with a stable, pain-free, plantigrade foot. Revisional hindfoot surgery is considered a salvage procedure and all risks involved, including infection, nonunion, or limb loss, must be discussed at length with the patient. The extended convalescence period is also a factor. Most often the postoperative treatment protocol is more emotionally and physically stressful to the patient than the surgical intervention itself.

During this preliminary period of evaluation or in cases in which the patient is not a surgical candidate, bracing (including Charcot restraint orthotic walker, ankle-foot orthosis) or other devices (including electric and ultrasonic bone stimulators) can be implemented.

SURGICAL TECHNIQUES

Infection

Before any definitive arthrodesis procedure, any infectious process must be eradicated. If advanced imaging was inconclusive, bone biopsy and culture should be performed. Retained hardware should also be removed at this time. Two patients treated at our institution presented with an infected lower extremity with a retained intramedullary rod. Because of the nature and placement of the rod, it must be considered that the medullary canal is part of the infectious process. After initial debridement of the infected tissue the retained hardware was removed and an antibiotic-impregnated bone cement rod replaced the implant. This rod was designed with use of a surgical chest tube and a 0.062 Kirschner wire for structure and placement (**Fig. 1**). Gentamicin was used as the antibiotic because of culture results and its heat-stable properties. This constant local delivery of antibiotics remained for approximately 10 weeks while the patient received 6 weeks of intravenous (IV) antibiotics. Supplemental external fixation was used in one case because of severe instability. Follow-up cultures were taken during the final revisional procedure and were found to be negative, resulting in the ability for the placement of internal hardware after removal of the polymethyl methacrylate (PMMA) rod for the final arthrodesis procedure.

Madanagopal and colleagues[46] in 2004 described a similar technique for treatment of infected tibial nails for tibial shaft fractures. Thonse and Conway[58] in 2007 demonstrated a 95% control of infection with the use of an antibiotic cement–coated interlocking intramedullary nail for treatment of various lower extremity infected nonunions. They advocated only removing the nail if infection or nonunion persisted. This procedure is a consideration for patients unwilling to have external fixation for supplemental stability if the arthrodesis site is too unstable for a temporary rod only.

Local antibiotic-impregnated bone cement can also be used for the initial treatment of large central defects created by extensive debridement of infected tissue. Recently a patient presented to our institution for a second opinion on a left ankle nonunion with a chronic draining sinus. After thorough evaluation and positive culture results, the patient was taken to the OR for extensive debridement, placement of an antibiotic-impregnated bone cement spacer, and application of an external fixator (**Fig. 2**). Working closely with our infective disease team, it was also agreed to send the patient home on

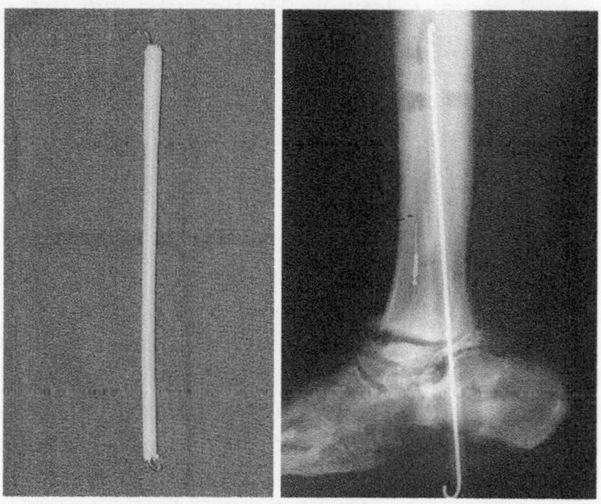

Fig. 1. For treatment of osteomyelitis with a retained intramedullary rod, an antibiotic-impregnated bone cement rod can be fashioned from a surgical test tube and 0.062 Kirschner wire. This design provides a constant local delivery of antibiotics after hardware removal and can coincide with long-term IV antibiotics. The rod is removed when the final revision is performed.

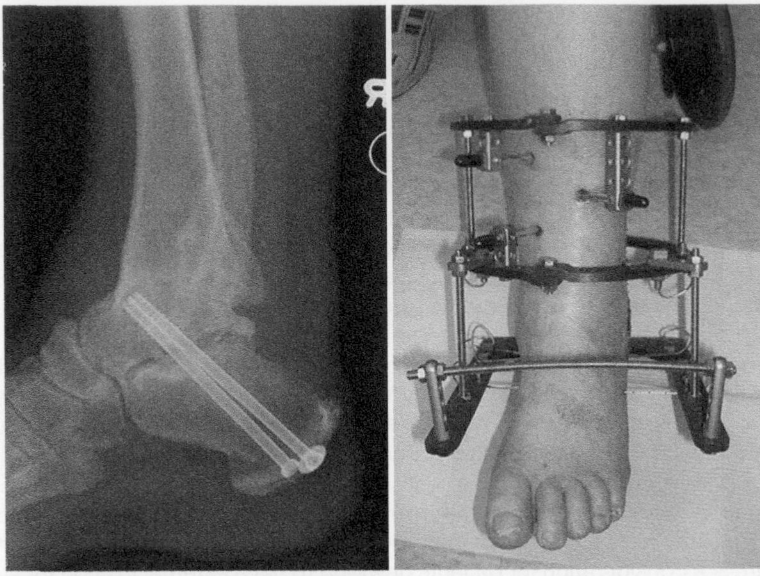

Fig. 2. This lateral radiograph demonstrates a subtalar nonunion, which was diagnosed with concomitant osteomyelitis. Original treatment consisted of extensive debridement, placement of antibiotic-impregnated bone cement, and external fixation for stability.

6 weeks of IV antibiotics. The patient further followed up for a staged tibiotalocalcaneal fusion after intraoperative cultures were negative.

Chan in 2000 and Chen in 2005 presented a staged treatment option for an infected tibial nonunion.[59,60] Initially the area was treated with thorough debridement and implantation of antibiotic-impregnated beads. Following a course of systemic antibiotics the fusion site was prepared with removal of the beads and placement of vancomycin-impregnated autogenic bone graft. Chan demonstrated a 98% union rate with a 92% infection arrest at 4 to 6 years' follow-up. He believed that this demonstrated that antibiotics impregnated into the graft had no adverse effects on bony incorporation and could be placed for supplemental local antibiotic coverage. Chen, however, had a 100% infection control with only a 72% bony fusion, thus leading to concerns of the impregnated antibiotic affecting bone graft incorporation.

Nonunion

Surgical intervention for a nonunion can be performed once all infection has been eliminated or ruled out. The type of arthrodesis to be performed must first be determined. Many times adjacent joints that were not fused with the initial surgery present with degeneration, pain, and decreased range of motion.[22,61] Previously attempted ankle fusions can present with extensive talar body destruction and require a tibiotalocalcaneal fusion for salvage.[62] At the authors' institution a previous patient had presented with chronic degenerative changes of the talonavicular joint due to a previous navicular fracture. A primary arthrodesis of the talonavicular joint was attempted. Postoperatively the patient developed a delayed union due to noncompliance with his nonweightbearing status and extensive tobacco use. Conservative treatment spanning the subsequent 11 months failed to heal the delayed union, which progressed to a nonunion. Follow-up radiographs also demonstrated increasing tritarsal joint changes. A triple arthrodesis was therefore performed with use of an iliac crest bone graft at the nonunion site. The patient went on to union with no major complications to date.

Considerations of hardware and incision placement must also be addressed. Various configurations have been described in literature and practiced at our institution. Katsenis and colleagues[63] in 2005 reported a 100% union rate in 21 patients treated with the Ilizarov method. Six were aseptic nonunions. Adjunct procedures included gradual distraction of a hypertrophic nonunion, tarsal tunnel release, Achilles tendon lengthening, and a proximal tibial osteotomy for limb lengthening. The most prevalent complications included pin site infections and axial deviation, which can be treated with frame modification. Other techniques of external fixation, including a Taylor spatial frame, for gradual correction of any malalignment have been discussed.[64–67] Midis and Conti[68] described the use of an external fixator for posttraumatic cases in which the skin remained tenuous and incision dehiscence or healing was a concern.

Intramedullary nails are only considered at our institution for use in a salvage procedure. Their use has been documented in the literature as a viable option for primary arthrodesis for patients who have severe deformities, rheumatoid arthritis, Charcot arthropathy, and avascular necrosis of the talus.[5,9,20,21,24,37,69] Documented complication rates include some greater than 50%, and excellent results are rare.[5,20,24,39,69]

With the stability of the construct and ability to use bone graft to surround the nail, this is a viable option for many patients who have extensive defects and poor bone quality (**Fig. 3**). Further literature supports these beliefs and other modifications for even greater stability. Chi and colleagues in 2001 described the use of a stainless steel semitubular plate on the lateral aspect of the calcaneus to supplement the original screw construct of the nail.[70] They found with revisional cases the lateral calcaneal wall was too soft for primary screws and washers. This construct allowed purchase of the screws without deformation into the calcaneus. Mader and colleagues in 2003 also confronted the issue of the calcaneal bone stock and questionable rotational stability of the intramedullary rod.[35] They proposed placing the rod in the posterior-anterior plane for placement of the distal calcaneal screws in this same

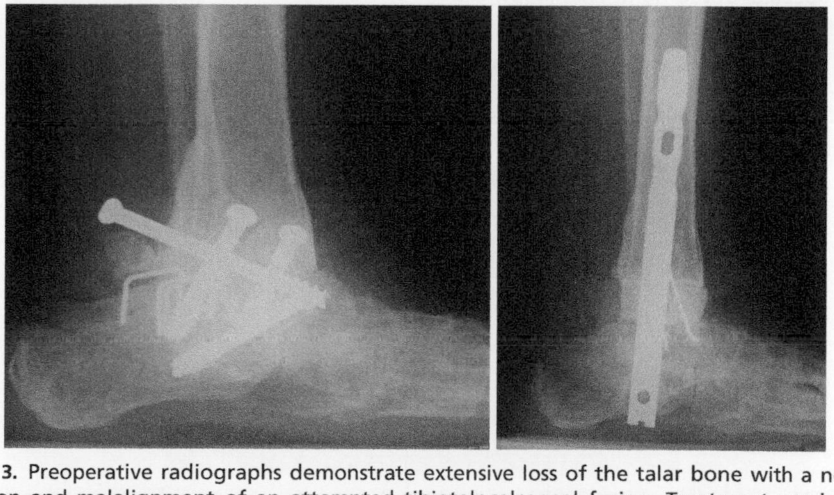

Fig. 3. Preoperative radiographs demonstrate extensive loss of the talar bone with a nonunion and malalignment of an attempted tibiotalocalcaneal fusion. Treatment consisted of a revisional tibiotalocalcaneal arthrodesis with allogenic fresh frozen femoral head bone graft and an intramedullary rod for fixation.

manner. They believed this provided better purchase on the bone and helped neutralize the sagittal forces at the fusion site.

Rigid internal fixation with the use of screws or plates should be considered in cases of adequate bone stock and soft tissue envelope. Documented fusion rates range from 72% to 94% for revisional cases of hindfoot arthrodeses. This fixation provides adequate compression and stabilization without the risk for pin tract infections or unwanted compression on adjacent joints.[22,61,71]

The necessity for bone graft material in a primary hindfoot arthrodesis remains controversial; however, it is considered standard of care for revisional procedures.[31] Autograft, allograft, and bone graft substitutes, including demineralized bone matrix (DBM), autologous platelet concentrate, and coralline hydroxyapatite, have been described for use in lower extremity fusions (**Fig. 4**).[27,72–86]

Autogenic bone graft is the only graft material that currently can provide all three characteristics of bone healing. Osteoconduction, osteoinduction, and osteogenesis provide an exceptional environment for bone healing. Multiple reports in literature support the belief that autogenic bone graft is superior in revisional surgery.[72,75,76,78,83,87] Harvest sites include anterior and posterior iliac crest, anterior tibia, fibula, and calcaneus.[75,76,78,81,84,86,87] At our institution, nonunions requiring joint debridement and angular deformity correction are supplemented with autogenic bone graft material. Local fibular bone graft often times is used with revisional ankle fusions either as morselized bone graft material or as an onlay structural graft. Cancellous grafting needed only for its osteoinductive properties can be harvested from local sites in the lower extremity.[76,83,84] When a large structural graft is needed, iliac crest is harvested for us by our orthopedic or plastic surgeons. Complication rates range from 0.5% to 10% for iliac crest bone graft harvest.[31,88–90] Ailments of long-term pain, seroma, hematoma, neuroma, infection, fracture, and hernia have all lead to the use of substitutes, thus leading to less morbidity and perceived equivalent success.[31,88–90] Bishop and colleagues[78] in 1995 presented a case study of 11 patients who had a large residual bone defect at the ankle level due to infection, tumor, trauma, or nonunion. Treatment consisted of the use of a free vascularized autogenic bone graft from the fibula for defects larger than 4 cm and iliac crest for smaller defects. Nine out of 11 patients had a successful outcome at final follow-up.

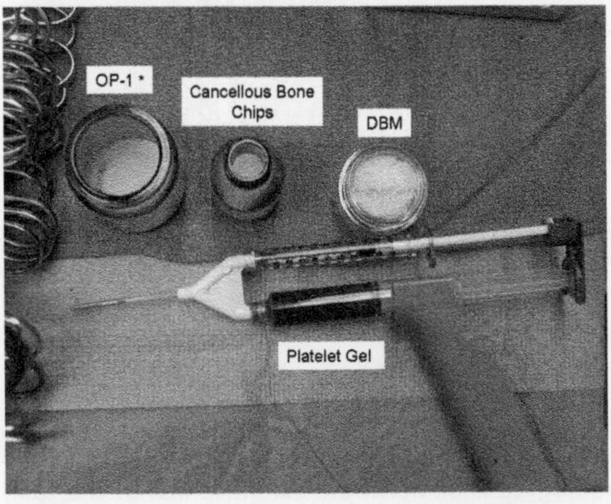

Fig. 4. Various bone graft materials and substitutes can be used to enhance revisional arthrodesis sites, including autologous platelet concentrate, DBM, OP-1, and various other products.

Results of revisional hindfoot arthrodesis with use of allograft alone have been poor with a significant number of residual nonunions.[5,22,73] Large defects resulting from extensive osseous débridements have limited options, however. With these salvage cases structural allograft may be considered.[5] At our institution cases involving extensive evacuation of infected or avascular bone may times result in the need for fresh frozen allograft. Placement of a femoral head within the cavity provides the structure and osteoconduction needed. We complement this with bone graft substitutes and local autogenic bone graft to provide the necessary osteoinduction and osteogenesis for superior results.

Synthetic bone graft substitutes, bone morphogenetic proteins (BMPs), DBM, autologous platelet concentrate, and bone marrow aspirate are all adjunct therapies that can be considered for revisional hindfoot arthrodeses. Calcium-based ceramic bone graft substitutes can be combined with autogenic cancellous graft to provide an osteoconductive bone void filler. There are no data to date to support the use of these materials alone to treat nonunions.[72]

BMPs, specifically BMP-2 and -7, possess osteoinductive activity that has been developed for clinical use.[72] The downfall of this material is that it requires 10 to 1000 times greater amount in humans compared with animal models to elicit this response. Further investigation into protein and gene therapy is therefore evolving to prolong the level of effective BMP in the human body.[72] Currently BMP is implanted through a collagen-based carrier, which provides osteoconduction at the same site. Several studies have been presented on fusion rates with BMP-7 (also known as osteogenic protein-1 [OP-1; Stryker Biotech, Hopkinton, Massachusetts]) for spinal fusions in animal and human studies.[91–95] Johnsson and colleagues compared the use of autograft bone (iliac crest) versus OP-1 for posterolateral spinal fusions in a patient population of 20. They concluded that there was no significant difference between the study groups at 1 year follow-up.[91] Vaccaro and colleagues[93] in 2003 presented a study on the safety and efficacy of OP-1 as an adjunct to iliac crest autograft to posterolateral lumbar fusions in 12 patients. Complete fusion was only reported in 55% of the population; however, improvement in symptoms was noted in 75%. This finding is slightly greater than the documented 45% fusion rate with allograft alone while demonstrating no adverse effects with the use of OP-1.

Currently OP-1 is approved by the US Food and Drug Administration (FDA) for treatment of nonunions in long bones. OP-1 has been shown to be equivalent or greater in success than autograft alone.[94] Fusion rate of 89% after previous failure with use of iliac bone graft has been published while following the treatment protocol for long bone nonunions consisting of OP-1, local bone graft, and stable fixation. At our institution we follow this same regimen in revisional nonunion cases. Many times we have combined the OP-1 with local fibular graft for interposition at ankle fusion sites. This procedure can be in adjunct with a femoral head allograft for larger defects. Our early results have been promising in revisional tibiotalocalcaneal fusions and Charcot reconstructions.

Autologous platelet concentrate and DBM are also advocated for use as adjunct therapies in revisional fusions of the hindfoot at our institution. Autologous platelet concentrate provides an increased amount of growth factor at the surgical site, which in turn has demonstrated the ability to induce bone formation.[80,96] DBM, which is derived from processed cortical bone, displays various amounts of osteoconductive and osteoinductive properties.[72] Research has been presented on equal healing rates and time to fusion using DBM versus iliac crest autograft in primary hindfoot arthrodesis.[27] There are no clinical trials on its use alone for revisional fusions to date, however.

Adequate joint preparation and proper alignment are essential for a satisfactory outcome. Adjunct surgical procedures, including posterior muscle group lengthening, nerve decompression, and forefoot reconstruction, may be necessary during the reconstruction.

Supplemental treatment of hindfoot nonunions includes the use of an electric bone stimulator. This treatment may be invasive, semi-invasive, or evasive. We prefer implantable bone stimulators when indicated because of the inconsistent patient compliance with external stimulators and continual direct current on the fusion site. Pulsing electromagnetic field therapy has been FDA approved for stimulation of bone growth for failed arthrodesis.[97] Recent literature specifically focusing on hindfoot arthrodesis has had various results for treatment of primary fusions or delayed unions.[97,98] Two studies on implantable electric bone stimulation with surgical hindfoot arthrodesis for high-risk hindfoot fusions demonstrated fusion rates of 86% to 92%.[99,100] The greatest complication, although small, was irritation by the battery pack, which resulted in removal in a small number of patients. Bassett and colleagues presented an 82% fusion rate in 71 cases of failed arthrodeses and therefore advocated the use of a bone stimulator in adjunct with further surgical treatment when necessary.[101] Midis and Conti[68] in 2002 presented a 100% fusion rate in 10 patients who had a revisional ankle fusion with use of external fixation, bone graft, and an implantable bone stimulator.

Exogenous ultrasound for bone stimulation is an alternative to electric bone stimulation. Low-intensity exogenous ultrasound is indicated for nonunions and it used in 20-minute intervals daily verses 10 to 12 hours needed for electric bone stimulators. Jones and colleagues[102] in 2006 reported on 13 revisional hindfoot arthrodesis procedures performed with adjunct ultrasonic therapy. Based on CT scans there was a 65% union rate (13 unions) with 5 partial unions and 1 nonunion. Exogenous ultrasound is also an adjunctive therapy that can be considered.

Malunion

At our institution we have found that patients primarily present with either a valgus or varus malposition of their hindfoot with additional rotation or anterior translation (**Fig. 5**), which in turn causes increased stress on adjacent joints and soft tissues, leading to increased disability and pain.[40] Primary surgical malalignment and fixed compensatory contractures must be uncovered and treated. Incision placement, surgical technique, and fixation are all dictated through the initial findings. Evaluation of appropriate radiographs demonstrates where the CORA lies and which approach is necessary for proper realignment.

Hindfoot alignment

At the Western Pennsylvania Hospital, we rely on optimal realignment of the hindfoot for success and this has a few key aspects that always need to be addressed. They are as follows: (1) the foot is at a right angle to the leg (mid-diaphyseal line of the tibia and the plantar aspect of the foot) and the tibia mid-diaphyseal line coincides with the lateral process of the talus in the sagittal plane, (2) the foot is slightly externally rotated with respect to the leg in the transverse plane (the tibial tuberosity should coincide with the longitudinal axis of the second digit) so that the talo–first metatarsal angle is aligned parallel, and (3) the relation of the mid-diaphyseal line of the tibia to the calcaneal bisection line should be parallel to 2° valgus and 5 to 10 mm lateral in the frontal plane.[51] This evaluation should be used with all types of hindfoot arthrodesis procedures for optimal results.

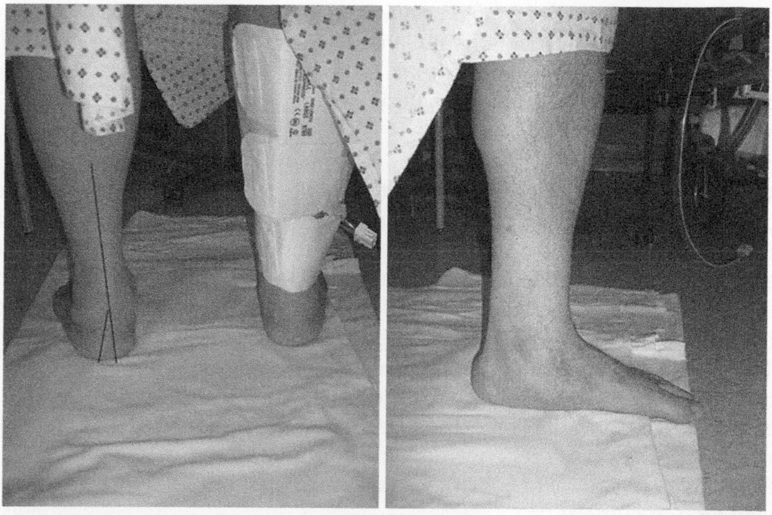

Fig. 5. Malunions often present with residual varus, valgus or rotational deformities. The patient presented with left foot chronic medial arch and lateral column pain after undergoing a triple arthrodesis with residual valgus malalignment.

Ankle malunion

Research on supramalleolar osteotomies for distal tibial deformities and malunion ankle arthrodeses have been published with promising results.[61,63,103–106] These procedures can performed as wedge cuts, straight cuts, or focal dome osteotomies.[103] When planning, the focal dome can rotate through its axis, whereas the straight and wedge osteotomies may also need translation to provide accurate realignment. This need can be minimalized by performing the osteotomy as near to the CORA as possible. Internal or external fixation may be warranted in these cases depending on the patient's size, ability to be nonweightbearing, and extent of correction needed. Gradual correction may be warranted if the soft tissue structures are contracted.

Focal dome osteotomies also provide the ability for posterior placement of the foot on the ankle. Anterior translation is often seen in painful nonunions with the patient's primary complaint of midfoot pain attributable to the overloading of these joints.[61] Posterior translation of the foot with the talar lateral process coinciding with the mid-diaphyseal line of the tibia reduces the length of that anterior lever arm of the foot and provides a mechanical advantage during the stance phase of gait.[63]

A slight limb shortening on the affected side, which may occur because of the surgical procedure, is not always detrimental and can facilitate toe clearance during the swing phase of gait.[63,107]

Anterior-posterior, lateral, and long leg calcaneal axial views can be performed in the OR under image intensification to assess sagittal, transverse, and frontal planes.[51,52] It is imperative that the foot is loaded to simulate weightbearing to allow proper evaluation of the osseous segments and their alignment.

Casillas and Allen[106] in 2004 presented their own classification system for treatment of malunion ankle arthrodeses, including wedge osteotomies and various fixation devices with concomitant triple arthrodeses in select cases of hindfoot arthritis with a fixed deformity. Cooper[39] in 2001 presented a similar algorithm for failed ankle arthrodeses and Anderson and colleagues[61] presented a direct technique of an osteotomy through the previous fusion site with realignment and screw fixation resulting in a plantigrade limb in all but one patient at final follow-up.[39,61] The one malunion was a residual varus deformity with chronic pain. This deformity has been well documented as a less tolerable or compensated position than residual valgus.

Rearfoot malunion

Evaluation of the hindfoot and forefoot must be performed when considering the type and location of the arthrodesis. If the deformity lies in the hindfoot alone a revisional subtalar joint fusion could be considered. If any deformity also lies within the midfoot, however, a triple arthrodesis should be considered to help realign the entire foot.[108]

In situ subtalar joint arthrodeses or revisional bone block arthrodeses can be performed to align the talo–first metatarsal angle and hindfoot varus or valgus. If this is not sufficient, a calcaneal osteotomy may be performed with medial or lateral translation with or without a possible wedge to reduce this deformity (**Fig. 6**).[108] With a varus hindfoot, excessive plantarflexion of the first ray may be present and exaggerated with realignment. Always take into consideration the unmasking or worsening of such deformities during realignment, which should be addressed with a dorsiflexory osteotomy at the time of surgery.[108]

If a patient presents with adjacent joint degeneration or a previous triple arthrodesis has been performed with residual deformity remaining, than a revisional triple arthrodesis may indicated. Many surgical approaches to this arthrodesis have been presented in the literature, all with the same goal of a plantigrade limb. Pomeroy and Manoli[108] in 1996 described direct osteotomies within the previous fusion sites with rotation and translation of the hindfoot for realignment. With residual forefoot deformities they recommended dialing down the supinatus through the talonavicular and calcaneocuboid joints or a plantarflexory osteotomy of the first ray for residual pronation. Toolan[109] in 2004 described a technique of a biplanar, opening-closing wedge osteotomy of the midfoot for correction of painful rockerbottom deformity after a maligned triple arthrodesis. This technique lead to less bony resection and therefore less shortening of the foot compared with other surgical techniques. Haddad and colleagues[110] in 1997 proposed an algorithmic approach to revisional surgery for failed triple arthrodesis. This approach was based on the type and extent of hindfoot deformity present and any concomitant forefoot deformity.

If adjacent ankle arthritis is present because of longstanding deformity and compensation, a revised triple arthrodesis with an ankle fusion or total ankle replacement may be indicated (**Fig. 7**).[108] Internal fixation or retrograde intramedullary rodding may be indicated in specific cases.

If significant hindfoot valgus is present, consideration of incision placement becomes essential. With a large acute correction, skin tension on traditional laterally based incisions result in wound dehiscence or soft tissue complications.[69] This result can be prevented through either a medial approach and acute correction or gradual correction with use of external fixation. Jackson and colleagues[45] in 2007 described a medial-approach triple arthrodesis for correction of eight feet with severe hindfoot valgus. There were no primary wound dehiscences, with a mean time to arthrodesis of 5.25 months. Rush[111] in 2007 also described the use of a medial hindfoot incision for malunion associated with flatfoot procedures. This procedure avoided lateral soft tissue adaptation and greater access to the middle and anterior facets of the subtalar joint.

Adjunctive soft tissue procedures, including peroneal tendon lengthening, posterior muscle group lengthening, and posterior tibial tendon repair with associated tendon transfers, should be performed when indicated.

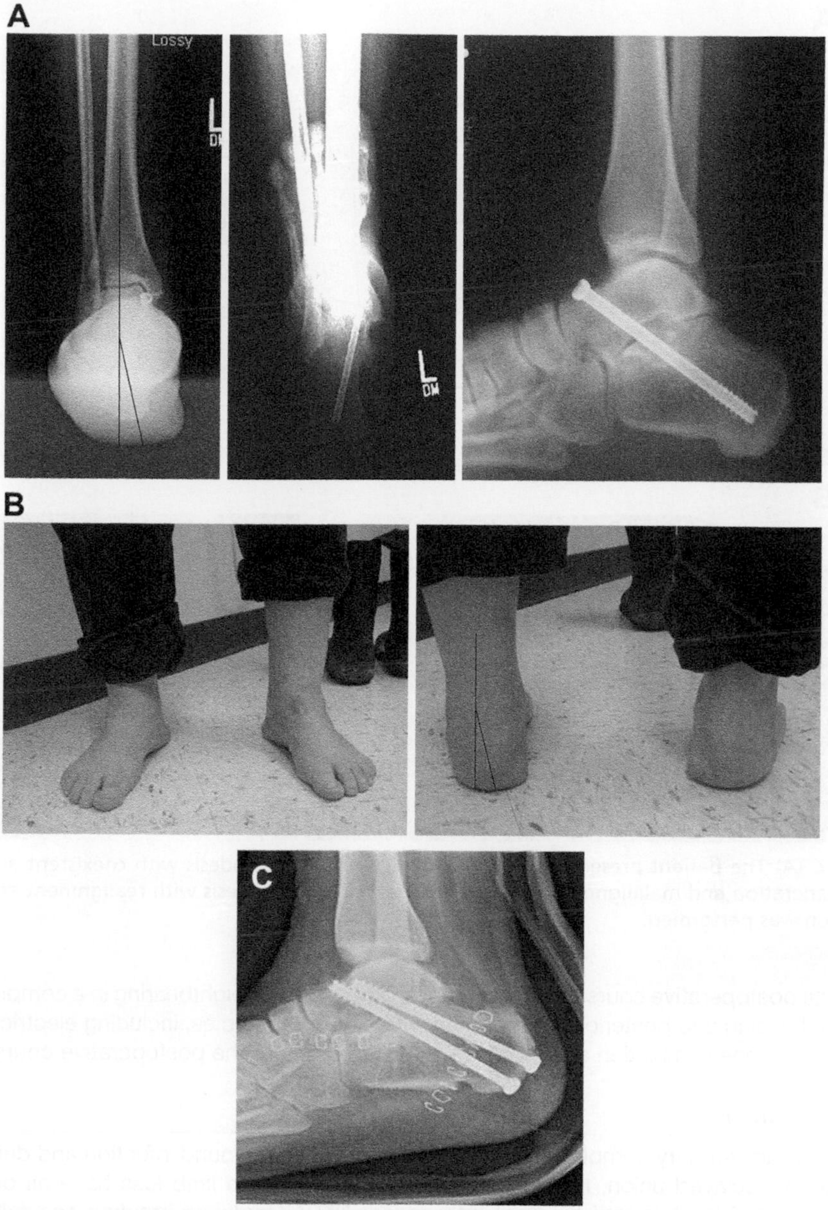

Fig. 6. (*A*) Preoperative radiographs, including long leg calcaneal axial and hindfoot alignment films, demonstrate a subtalar nonunion with varus malalignment. (*B*) Clinically, the patient complained of lateral column overload and chronic ankle sprains. (*C*) A revisional subtalar arthrodesis with a posterior calcaneal osteotomy was performed for satisfactory realignment with two screws to increase stability.

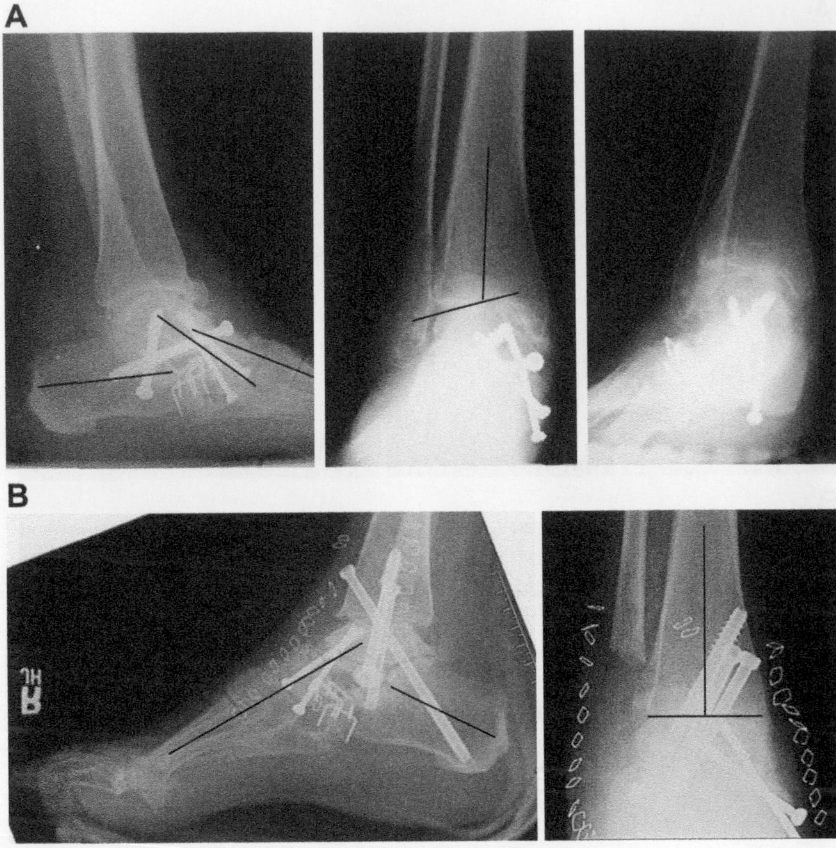

Fig. 7. (*A*) The patient presented with a nonunion triple arthrodesis with coexistent ankle degeneration and malalignment. (*B*) A revisional triple arthrodesis with realignment ankle fusion was performed.

The postoperative course should include complete nonweightbearing in a compression dressing and posterior splint or cast with adjunct therapies, including electric/ultrasonic bone stimulation and close follow-up throughout the postoperative course.

Complications

As with any surgery complications can occur. Superficial wound infection and dehiscence to delayed union, nonunion, residual malunion, and limb loss have all been documented in revisional hindfoot arthrodeses.[40,112] Hardware irritation and failure are among the most frequent reasons to return to the OR. Thomas and colleagues[107] in 2006 evaluated the gait disturbances in patients who had received an ankle arthrodesis. They found substantial differences in hindfoot function and gait compared with a normal population. They expressed the importance of communication with patients about the extent of the salvage procedure, which subsequently causes persistent alterations in gait. Mitchell and colleagues in 1995 presented three cases of associated tibial stress fractures following pantalar fusions.[113] As with any salvage procedure, the complications can be great and have been reported as high as 50% in revisional hindfoot arthrodeses.[20,69]

SUMMARY

Salvage of a failed hindfoot arthrodesis is an extensive undertaking for the surgeon and patient. Time to fusion for revisional hindfoot surgery ranges from 8 weeks to 6 months compared with primary hindfoot arthrodesis of 47 days to 4 months.[1,16,33,36,61,110] With increased morbidity and postoperative convalescence and complications, patients must understand the risk involved in this type of revisional surgery. Preoperative evaluation, accurate surgical technique, adequate fixation, and intraoperative alignment, are all essential for a successful outcome.

REFERENCES

1. Ferkel R, Hewitt M. Long-term results of arthroscopic ankle arthrodesis. Foot Ankle Int 2005;26(4):275–80.
2. Talarico L, Vito G. Triple arthrodesis using external ring fixation and arched-wire compression. JAPMA 2004;94(1):12–21.
3. Donatto K. Arthritis and arthrodesis of the hindfoot. Clin Orthop Relat Res 1998; 349:81–92.
4. Ahmad J, Pour A, Raikin S. The modified use of a proximal humeral locking plate for tibiotalcalcaneal arthrodesis. Foot Ankle Int 2007;28(9):977–83.
5. Pelton K, Hofer J, Thordarson D. Tibiotalocalcaneal arthrodesis using a dynamically locked retrograde intramedullary nail. Foot Ankle Int 2006;27(10):759–63.
6. Haskell A, Pfeiff C, Mann R. Subtalar joint arthrodesis using a single lag screw. Foot Ankle Int 2004;25(11):774–7.
7. Davies M, Rosenfeld P, Stavrou P, et al. A comprehensive review of subtalar arthrodesis. Foot Ankle Int 2007;28(3):295–7.
8. Bennett G, Cameron B, Njus G, et al. Tibiotalocalcaneal arthrodesis: a biomechanical assessment of stability. Foot Ankle Int 2005;26(7):530–6.
9. Chou L, Mann R, Yaszay B, et al. Tibiotalocalcaneal arthrodesis. Foot Ankle Int 2000;21(10):804–8.
10. Catanzariti A, Mendicino R, Saltrick K, et al. Subtalar joint arthrodesis. JAPMA 2005;95(1):34–41.
11. Castro M. Arthrodesis of the navicular. Foot Ankle Clin N Am 2004;9:73–83.
12. Alfahd U, Roth S, Stephen D, et al. Biomechanical comparison of intramedullary nail and blade plate fixation for tibiotalocalcaneal arthrodesis. J Orthop Trauma 2005;19(10):703–8.
13. Mandracchia V, Nickles W, Mandi D, et al. Treatment of nonunited hindfoot fusions. Clin Podiatr Med Surg 2004;21:417–39.
14. Papa J, Myerson M, Girard P. Salvage, with arthrodesis, in intractable diabetic neuropathic arthropathy of the foot and ankle. J Bone Joint Surg Am 1993; 75-A(7):1056–66.
15. Caron M, Kron E, Saltrick K. Tibiotalar joint arthrodesis for the treatment of severe ankle joint degeneration secondary to rheumatoid arthritis. Clin Podiatr Med Surg 1999;16(2):337–61.
16. Collman D, Kaas M, Schuberth J. Arthroscopic ankle arthrodesis: factors influencing union in 39 consecutive patients. Foot Ankle Int 2006;27(12):1079–85.
17. Huang P, Fu Y, Lu C, et al. Hindfoot arthrodesis for neuropathic deformity. Kaohsiung J Med Sci 2007;23(3):120–6.
18. Anderson T, Maxander P, Rydholm U, et al. Ankle arthrodesis by compression screws in rheumatoid arthritis: primary nonunion in 9/35 patients. Acta Orthop 2005;76(6):884–90.

19. Acosta R, Ushiba J, Cracchiolo A. The results of a primary and staged pantalar arthrodesis and tibiotalocalcaneal arthrodesis in adult patients. Foot Ankle Int 2000;21(3):182–94.
20. Mendicino R, Catanzariti A, Saltrick K, et al. Tibiotalocalcaneal arthrodesis with retrograde intramedullary nailing. J Foot Ankle Surg 2004;43(2):82–6.
21. Hammett R, Hepple S, Forster B, et al. Tibiotalocalcaneal arthrodesis by retrograde intramedullary nailing using a curved locking nail. The results of 52 procedures. Foot Ankle Int 2005;26(10):810–5.
22. Easely M, Trnka H, Schon L, et al. Isolated subtalar arthrodesis. J Bone Joint Surg 2005;82-A(5):613–24.
23. Trnka H, Easely M, Lam P, et al. Subtalar distraction bone block arthrodesis. J Bone Joint Surg Br 2001;83-B(6):849–54.
24. Niinimaki T, Klemola T, Leppilahti J. Tibiotalocalcaneal arthrodesis with a compressive retrograde intramedullary nail: a report of 34 consecutive patients. Foot Ankle Int 2007;28(4):431–4.
25. Miehlke W, Gschwend N, Rippstein P, et al. Compression arthrodesis of the rheumatoid ankle and hindfoot. Clin Orthop Relat Res 1997;340:75–86.
26. Perlman M, Thordarson D. Ankle fusion in a high risk population: an assessment of nonunion risk factors. Foot Ankle Int 1999;20(8):491–6.
27. Michelson J, Curl L. Use of demineralized bone matrix in hindfoot arthrodesis. Clin Orthop Relat Res 1996;325:203–8.
28. Saltzman C, Fehrle M, Cooper R, et al. Triple arthrodesis: twenty-five and forty-four-year average follow-up of the same patients. J Bone Joint Surg Am 1999; 81-A(10):1391–402.
29. Buchner M, Sabo D. Ankle fusion attributable to posttraumatic arthrosis: a long-term followup of 48 patients. Clin Orthop Relat Res 2003;406:155–64.
30. Smith R, Wood P. Arthrodesis of the ankle in the presence of a large deformity in the coronal plane. J Bone Joint Surg Br 2007;89-B(5):615–9.
31. Rosenfeld P, Budgen S, Saxby T. Triple arthrodesis: is bone grafting necessary. J Bone Joint Surg Br 2005;87-B(2):175–8.
32. Galindo M, Siff S, Butler J, et al. Triple arthrodesis in young children: a salvage procedure after failed releases in severely affected feet. Foot Ankle 1987;7(6): 319–25.
33. Mann R, Rongstad K. Arthrodesis of the ankle: a critical analysis. Foot Ankle Int 1998;19(1):3–9.
34. Takakura Y, Tanaka Y, Sugimoto K, et al. Long term results of arthrodesis for osteoarthritis of the ankle. Clin Orthop Relat Res 1999;361:178–85.
35. Mader K, Pennig D, Gausepohl T, et al. Calcaneotalotibial arthrodesis with a retrograde posterior-to-anterior locked nail as a salvage procedure for severe ankle pathology. J Bone Joint Surg Am 2003;85-A(4):123–8.
36. Wera G, Sontich J. Tibiotalar arthrodesis using a custom blade plate. J Trauma 2007;63(6):1279–82.
37. Anderson T, Linder L, Rydholm U, et al. Tibio-talocalcaneal arthrodesis as a primary procedure using a retrograde intramedullary nail. Acta Orthop 2005;76(4): 580–7.
38. Berend M, Glisson R, Nunley J. A biomechanical comparison of intramedullary nail and crossed lag screw fixation for tibiotalocalcaneal arthrodesis. Foot Ankle Int 1997;18(10):639–43.
39. Cooper P. Complications of ankle and tibiotalocalcaneal arthrodesis. Clin Orthop Relat Res 2001;391:33–44.

40. Van Bergeyk A, Stotler W, Beals T, et al. Functional outcome after modified Blair tibiotalar arthrodesis for talar osteonecrosis. Foot Ankle Int 2003;24(10):765–70.
41. Scranton P. Comparison of open isolated subtalar arthrodesis with autogenous bone graft versus outpatient arthroscopic subtalar arthrodesis using injectable bone morphogenic protein-enhanced graft. Foot Ankle Int 1999;20(3):162–5.
42. Jeray K, Rentz J, Ferguson R. Local bone-graft technique for subtalar extraarticular arthrodesis in cerebral palsy. J Pediatr Orthop 1998;18(1):75–80.
43. Ebraheim N, Elgafy H, Stefancin J. Intramedullary fibular graft for tibiotalocalcaneal arthrodesis. Clin Orthop Relat Res 2001;385:165–9.
44. Massari L, Gildone A, Zerbinati F. Tibiotalocalcaneal arthrodesis by retrograde intramedullary nailing as a salvage procedure: clinical, radiographic and baropodometric evaluation of three cases. Foot Ankle Surg 2002;8:3–12.
45. Jackson W, Tryfonidis M, Cooke P, et al. Arthrodesis of the hindfoot for valgus deformity. An entirely medial approach. J Bone Joint Surg Br 2007;89-B(7):925–7.
46. Madanagopal S, Seligson D, Roberts C. The antibiotic cement nail for infection after tibial nailing. Orthopedics 2004;27(7):709–12.
47. Ishikawa S, Murphy A, Richardson G. The effect of cigarette smoking on hindfoot fusions. Foot Ankle Int 2002;23(11):996–8.
48. Maenpaa H, Lehto M, Belt E. Why do ankle arthrodeses fail in patients with rheumatic disease. Foot Ankle Int 2001;22(5):403–8.
49. Kwiatkowski T, Hanley E, Ramp W. Cigarette smoking and its orthopedic consequences. Am J Orthop 1996;9:590–7.
50. Jensen J, Jensen T, Smith T, et al. Nutrition in orthopaedic surgery. J Bone Joint Surg Am 1982;64-A(9):1263–72.
51. Mendicino R, Lamm B, Catanzariti A, et al. Realignment arthrodesis of the rearfoot and ankle. JAPMA 2005;95(1):60–71.
52. Mendicino R, Catanzariti A, John S, et al. Long leg calcaneal axial and hindfoot alignment. Radiographic views for frontal plane assessment. JAPMA 2008; 98(1):75–8.
53. Mendicino R, Catanzariti A, Reeves C, et al. A systematic approach to evaluation of the rearfoot, ankle, and leg in reconstructive surgery. JAPMA 2005;95(1): 2–12.
54. Catanzariti A, Mendicino R, Whitaker J, et al. Realignment considerations in the triple arthrodesis. JAPMA 2005;95(1):13–7.
55. Lamm B, Mendicino B, Catanzariti A, et al. Static rearfoot alignment. A comparison of clinical and radiographic measures. JAPMA 2005;95(1):26–33.
56. Lamm B, Paley D. Deformity correction planning for hindfoot, ankle, and lower limb. Clin Podiatr Med Surg 2004;21:305–26.
57. Johnson J, Lamdan R, Granberry W, et al. Hindfoot coronal alignment: a modified radiographic method. Foot Ankle Int 1999;20(12):818–25.
58. Thonse R, Conway J. Antibiotic cement-coated interlocking nail for the treatment of infected nonunions and segmental bone defects. J Orthop Trauma 2007; 21(4):258–68.
59. Chan Y, Wen-Neng S, Wang C, et al. Antibiotic-impregnated autogenic cancellous bone grafting is an effective and safe method for the management of small infected tibial defects: a comparison study. J Trauma 2000;48(2):246–55.
60. Chen C, Ko J, Pan C. Results of vancomycin-impregnated cancellous bone grafting for infected tibial nonunion. Arch Orthop Trauma Surg 2005;125:369–75.
61. Anderson J, Coetzee C, Hansen S. Revision ankle fusion using internal compression arthrodesis with screw fixation. Foot Ankle Int 1997;18(5):300–9.

62. Edelman R, Fisher G. Tibiocalcaneal arthrodesis of a failed ankle fusion. J Foot Ankle Surg 1993;32(2):197–203.
63. Katsenis D, Bhave A, Paley D, et al. Treatment of malunion and nonunion at the site of an ankle fusion with the Ilizarov apparatus. J Bone Joint Surg 2005;87:302–9.
64. Zarutsky E, Rush S, Schuberth J. The use of circular wire external fixation in the treatment of salvage ankle arthrodesis. J Foot Ankle Surg 2005;44(1):22–31.
65. Newman A. Ankle fusion with the Hoffmann external fixation device. Foot Ankle 1980;1(2):102–9.
66. Feldman D, Shin S, Madan S, et al. Correction of tibial malunion and nonunion with six-axis analysis deformity correction using the Taylor spatial frame. J Orthop Trauma 2003;17(8):549–54.
67. Laughlin R, Calhoun J. Ring fixators for reconstruction of traumatic disorders of the foot and ankle. Orthop Clin North Am 1995;26(2):287–94.
68. Midis N, Conti S. Revision ankle arthrodesis. Foot Ankle Int 2002;23(3):243–7.
69. Millett P, O'Malley M, Tolo E, et al. Tibiotalocalcaneal fusion with a retrograde intramedullary nail: clinical and functional outcomes. Am J Orthop 2002;9:531–6.
70. Chi T, McWilliam J, Gould J. Lateral plate-washer technique for revision tibiocalcaneal fusion. Am J Orthop 2001;7:588–90.
71. Cheng Y, Chen S, Chen J, et al. Revision of ankle arthrodesis. Foot Ankle Int 2003;24(4):321–5.
72. Toolan B. Current concepts review: orthobiologics. Foot Ankle Int 2006;27(7): 561–6.
73. Bishop G, Einhorn T. Current and future clinical applications of bone morphogenetic proteins in orthopaedic trauma surgery. Int Orthop 2007;31:721–7.
74. McGarvey W, Braly W. Bone graft in hindfoot arthrodesis: allograft vs autograft. Orthopedics 1996;19(5):389–94.
75. Mahan K, Hillstrom H. Bone grafting in foot and ankle surgery. JAPMA 1998; 88(3):109–18.
76. Raikin S, Brislin K. Local bone graft harvested from the distal tibia or calcaneus for surgery of the foot and ankle. Foot Ankle Int 2005;26(6):449–53.
77. Scranton P Jr. Use of bone graft substitutes in lower extremity reconstructive surgery. Foot Ankle Int 2002;23(8):689–92.
78. Bishop A, Wood M, Sheetz K. Arthrodesis of the ankle with a free vascularized autogenous bone graft. Reconstruction of segmental loss of bone secondary to osteomyelitis, tumor, or trauma. J Bone Joint Surg Am 1995;77-A(12):1867–75.
79. Coetzee J, Pomeroy G, Watts J, et al. The use of autologous concentrated growth factors to promote syndesmosis fusion in the agility total ankle replacement. A preliminary study. Foot Ankle Int 2005;26(10):840–6.
80. Barrow C, Pomeroy G. Enhancement of syndesmotic fusion rates in total ankle arthroplasty with the use of autologous platelet concentrate. Foot Ankle Int 2005;26(6):458–61.
81. Geideman W, Early J, Brodsky J. Clinical results of harvesting autogenous cancellous graft from the ipsilateral proximal tibia for use in foot and ankle surgery. Foot Ankle Int 2004;25(7):451–5.
82. Coughlin M, Grimes J, Kennedy M. Coralline hydroxyapatite bone graft substitute in hindfoot surgery. Foot Ankle Int 2006;27(1):19–22.
83. Catanzariti A. Graft-enhanced arthrodesis. J Foot Ankle Surg 1996;35(5): 463–73.
84. Saltrick K, Caron M, Grossman J. Utilization of autogenous corticocancellous bone graft from the distal tibia for reconstructive surgery of the foot and ankle. J Foot Ankle Surg 1996;35(5):406–12.

85. Catanzariti A, Karlock L. The application of allograft bone in foot and ankle surgery. J Foot Ankle Surg 1996;35(5):440–51.
86. Storm T, Cohen J, Newton ED. Free vascularized bone graft. J Foot Ankle Surg 1996;35(5):436–9.
87. Mendicino R, Leonheart E, Shromoff P. Techniques for harvesting autogenous bone grafts of the lower extremity. J Foot Ankle Surg 1996;35(5):428–35.
88. DeOrio J, Farber D. Morbidity associated with anterior iliac crest bone grafting in foot and ankle surgery. Foot Ankle Int 2005;26(2):147–51.
89. Boone D. Complications of iliac crest graft and bone grafting alternatives in foot and ankle surgery. Foot Ankle Clin N Am 2003;8:1–14.
90. Tessier P, Kawamoto H, Posnick J, et al. Complications of harvesting autogenous bone grafts: a group experience of 20,000 cases. J Plast Recon Surg 2005;116(5):72S–3S.
91. Johnsson R, Stromqvist B, Aspenberg P. Randomized radiostereometric study comparing osteogenic protein-1 (BMP-7) and autograft bone in human noninstrumented posterolateral lumbar fusion. Spine 2002;27(23):2654–61.
92. Cunningham B, Kanayama M, Parker L, et al. Osteogenic protein versus autologous interbody arthrodesis in the sheep thoracic spine: a comparative endoscopic study using the Bagby and Kuslich interbody fusion device. Spine 1999;24(6):509–18.
93. Vaccaro A, Patel T, Fischgrund J, et al. A pilot safety and efficacy study of OP-1 putty as an adjunct to iliac crest autograft in posterolateral lumbar fusions. Eur Spine J 2003;12:495–500.
94. White A, Vaccaro A, Hall J, et al. Clinical applications of BMP-7/OP-1 in fractures, nonunions and spinal fusion. Int Orthop 2007;31:735–41.
95. Mont M, Jones L, Elias J, et al. Strut-autografting with and without osteogenic protein-1: a preliminary study of a canine femoral head defect model. J Bone Joint Surg 2001;83:1013–22.
96. Grant W, Jerlin E, Pietrzak W, et al. The utilization of autologous growth factors for the facilitation of fusion in complex neuropathic fractures in the diabetic population. Clin Podiatr Med Surg 2005;22:561–84.
97. Saltzman C, Lightfoot A, Amendola A. PEMF as treatment for delayed healing of foot and ankle arthrodesis. Foot Ankle Int 2004;25(11):771–3.
98. Dhawan S, Conti S, Towers J, et al. The effect of pulsed electromagnetic fields on hindfoot arthrodesis: a prospective study. J Foot Ankle Surg 2004;43(2):93–6.
99. Saxena A, DiDomenico L, Widtfeldt A, et al. Implantable electrical bone stimulation for arthrodeses of the foot and ankle in high-risk patients: A multicenter study. J Foot Ankle Surg 2005;44(6):450–4.
100. Donley B, Ward D. Implantable electrical stimulation in high-risk hindfoot fusions. Foot Ankle Int 2002;23(1):13–8.
101. Bassett C, Mitchell S, Gaston S. Pulsing electromagnetic field treatment in ununited fractures and failed arthrodeses. JAMA 1982;247(5):623–8.
102. Jones C, Coughlin M, Shurnas P. Prospective CT scan evaluation of hindfoot nonunions treated with revision surgery and low-intensity ultrasound stimulation. Foot Ankle Int 2006;27(4):229–35.
103. Mendicino R, Catanzariti A, Reeves C. Percutaneous supramalleolar osteotomy for distal tibial ankle deformities. JAPMA 2005;95(1):72–84.
104. Sen C, Kocaoglu M, Eralp L, et al. Correction of ankle and hindfoot deformities by supramalleolar osteotomy. Foot Ankle Int 2003;24(1):22–8.
105. Lubicky J, Altiok H. Transphyseal osteotomy of the distal tibia for correction of valgus/varus deformities of the ankle. J Pediatr Orthop 2001;21:80–8.

106. Casillas M, Allen M. Repair of malunions after ankle arthrodesis. Clin Podiatr Med Surg 2004;21:371–83.
107. Thomas R, Daniels T, Parker K. Gait analysis and functional outcomes following ankle arthrodesis for isolated ankle arthritis. J Bone Joint Surg Am 2006;88-A(3): 526–35.
108. Pomeroy G, Manoli A. Techniques of revision talocalcaneal arthrodesis. Tech Orthop 1996;11(4):347–54.
109. Toolan B. Revision of failed triple arthrodesis with an opening-closing wedge osteotomy of the midfoot. Foot Ankle Int 2004;25(7):456–61.
110. Haddad S, Myerson M, Pell R, et al. Clinical and radiographic outcome of revision surgery for failed triple arthrodesis. Foot Ankle Int 1997;18(8):489–99.
111. Rush S. Reconstructive options for failed flatfoot surgery. Clin Podiatr Med Surg 2007;24:779–88.
112. Maenpaa H, Lehto M, Belt E. What went wrong in triple arthrodesis. Clin Orthop Relat Res 2001;391:218–23.
113. Mitchell J, Johnson J, Collier D, et al. Stress fracture of the tibia following extensive hindfoot and ankle arthrodesis: a report of three cases. Foot Ankle Int 1995; 16(7):445–8.

Surgical Treatment of Calcaneal Fracture Malunions and Posttraumatic Deformities

John J. Stapleton, DPM, AACFAS[a], Ronald Belczyk, DPM, AACFAS[b], Thomas Zgonis, DPM, FACFAS[b,*]

KEYWORDS

- Revisional foot and ankle surgery • Complications
- Calcaneal fractures • Foot arthrodesis • Posttraumatic arthritis

The irregular contour of the calcaneus, the complexity of the mechanics of a three-facet subtalar joint, the surrounding neurovascular structures, and the delicate soft tissue envelope make operative intervention in this area a challenge fraught with possible complications. Many experienced surgeons acknowledge a steep and significant learning curve in the operative management of calcaneal fractures. Although controversy continues to surround this issue, nonoperative management of displaced intra-articular calcaneal fractures may result in malunion, thereby affecting the function of the ankle, subtalar, and transverse tarsal joints.[1] The primary fracture deformity contributes directly to late complications. Residual deformity and malunion after operative management of calcaneal fractures are a common reason for revisional surgery. The notion that Cotton and Henderson[2] stated in 1916 often holds some validity today that "ordinarily speaking, the man who breaks his heel bone is 'done' so far as his industrial future is concerned."

CALCANEAL MALUNIONS

Calcaneal malunions are problematic for several reasons.[1,3–14] Although some calcaneal fractures can be treated conservatively, a majority of them require operative

[a] Foot and Ankle Surgery, VSAS Orthopaedics, Allentown, PA, USA
[b] Department of Orthopaedics, Division of Podiatric Medicine and Surgery, The University of Texas Health Science Center at San Antonio, 7703 Floyd Curl Drive/ MCS 7776, San Antonio, TX 78229, USA
* Corresponding author.
E-mail address: zgonis@uthscsa.edu (T. Zgonis).

Clin Podiatr Med Surg 26 (2009) 79–90
doi:10.1016/j.cpm.2008.10.003

intervention to prevent functional impairment and disability, especially because most of these fractures affect young and middle-aged industrial workers.[12] Nonoperative management of these displaced fractures may result in a severely disabling fracture malunion that is associated with several typical findings that are discussed herein.

The calcaneus is the support for body weight from the initial heel contact with the ground reaction force to midstance during ambulation. The calcaneus supports the talus and its position in relation to the floor and determines the appropriate position of the articular surface of the talus with the tibia. The surface incongruity of the posterior subtalar facet joint over time results in painful posttraumatic arthritis. The lateral calcaneal wall expansion results in heel widening with associated subfibular impingement causing peroneal stenosis, tendinitis, or dislocation. The decrease in calcaneal body height results in loss of the talar declination which results in anterior tibiotalar impingement and diminished ankle range of motion. If the anterocalcaneal fracture extends into the calcaneal cuboid joint, resulting posttraumatic arthrosis can probably occur. A malunited calcaneal fracture tuberosity can result in varus hindfoot malalignment; therefore, the function of the ankle, subtalar, and transverse tarsal joints can all be affected, leading to pain and disability.

The surgeon needs to determine the reason for operative failure and whether revisional surgery would be beneficial to pursue. At times, revisional surgery can create further complications or increased pain leading to limb loss and in certain circumstances may need to be avoided. Understanding the common problems that can be successfully managed through revisional surgery is paramount to achieving reproducible and reasonable surgical outcomes.

Patient selection is essential to prevent postoperative complications, and the contraindications are the same as for initial surgical intervention of calcaneal fractures. With revisional calcaneal fracture surgery, the most common contraindication is usually a patient who should have not been operated on initially because of multiple comorbidities, active infection, or arterial insufficiency. A history of tobacco use has been shown to have detrimental effects on soft tissue healing and union rates. Smoking cessation needs to be enforced but is not usually a contraindication for revisional surgery.[12]

Revisional calcaneal fracture surgery is often indicated for infection, wound healing complications, deformity, malunion, nonunion, subtalar joint arthrosis, anterior ankle joint impingement, lateral ankle impingement, subluxation of the peroneal tendons, painful or broken hardware, sural neuritis, and tarsal tunnel syndrome. It is beyond the scope of this article to cover all facets of revisional surgery that can be associated with poor outcomes from operative intervention of calcaneal fractures.

Clinical and Radiographic Findings

Calcaneal fracture malunions affect the function of the ankle, subtalar, and calcaneal cuboid joints, eventually leading to pain or permanent disability. The initial patient evaluation for revisional surgery begins with a thorough clinical assessment of the factors that contribute to patient dissatisfaction, functional impairment, and pain. Posttraumatic subtalar and calcaneal cuboid arthrosis occurs secondary to residual articular incongruity. Anterior ankle impingement and loss of ankle dorsiflexion are complications from a loss in vertical height of the calcaneus. In addition, subfibular impingement results from a residual lateral wall expansion and heel widening. Frequently, the malunited calcaneal fracture involves some form of peroneal tendon pathology such as stenosis, subluxation, or dislocation. An altered and poorly tolerated gait pattern is secondary to a varus malunion of the calcaneal tuberosity.

Patients with a previous history of infection or wound healing complications present with an additional challenge to the treating physician. Elevations in the white blood cell count, sedimentation rate, and C-reactive protein increase the clinical suspicion for infection. If laboratory, clinical, or radiographic findings are suspicious for osteomyelitis, a white blood cell–labeled bone scan is performed in the absence of hardware or an indium 111–labeled bone scan in the presence of retained hardware. This study is often correlated with a bone marrow sulfur colloid scan and an MRI. If persistent infection is present, it is initially treated with debridement, bone biopsy, and hardware removal followed by external fixation methods for osseous and soft tissue stabilization, soft tissue coverage, and parenteral antibiotics based on intraoperative cultures.

Neurovascular injury can occur from the high-energy nature of the injury or resultant compartment syndrome. Patients with severe poorly localized pain should be evaluated for nerve-related problems and complex regional pain syndrome. A thorough neurologic examination should be performed in patients presenting with a calcaneal malunion. A late clinical presentation of claw toe deformities may be secondary to a missed compartment syndrome. Patients may complain of severe pain, sensory changes, and paresthesia along the tibial or sural nerve. Electrophysiologic testing may be warranted to assist in establishing the diagnosis and cause of pain along with lumbar sympathetic blocks if chronic pain syndromes are being considered. In these case scenarios, further surgical intervention should be delayed or coordinated with pain management specialists because reconstructive surgery alone will probably offer little relief in pain postoperatively.

Calcaneal varus deformities are commonly encountered when the medial face of the calcaneal wall has not been adequately reduced across the primary fracture line. Patients with a calcaneal varus deformity usually complain about lateral column pain, lateral ankle instability, or medial or lateral ankle joint pain. A thorough musculoskeletal examination should be performed. Physical examination can reveal a hindfoot varus deformity while the patient is standing. In some cases, the calcaneal tuberosity can appear rectus on examination while it remains in varus when evaluated radiographically with a hindfoot alignment view. This finding occurs in the presence of rearfoot edema or widening of the heel which masks the ability of the clinician to assess the true position of the calcaneal tuberosity. Ankle and subtalar range of motion should be assessed as well. Ankle joint dorsiflexion can be limited by tibiotalar exostosis or impingement secondary to an abnormal talar declination. Frequently, the subtalar joint remains stiff following a joint depression injury. Ankle instability can be checked with the anterior drawer and talar tilt tests clinically and radiographically. Gait examination may also reveal abnormalities with weakened push-off strength.

Radiographs are crucial in assessing calcaneal malunions. A lateral radiograph can reveal the degree of joint depression and loss of declination of the talus in relation to the floor. A decrease in calcaneal body height, as represented by a decreased or negative Bohler's angle, results in a more horizontal talus which, in turn, leads to anterior tibiotalar impingement and a decrease in ankle dorsiflexion. The surgeon also needs to evaluate the position of the calcaneal tuberosity on a standing hindfoot alignment view. Severe joint depression is usually the result of a "pulverized" calcaneal fracture, and the alignment of the tuberosity can be significantly placed in varus or valgus along with being translated medially or laterally. The bisection of the calcaneus on a hindfoot alignment view should be parallel to the anatomic axis of the distal tibia. The center of the calcaneus is approximately 5 to 10 mm lateral to the anatomic axis of the tibia. This position should be quantified through radiographs by performing standing hindfoot alignment views using the contralateral side as a control if unaffected. If bilateral calcaneal fractures are present, the surgeon should evaluate the deformity in relation to average normal parameters. Standing ankle views will determine if adaptive ankle joint deformity, arthrosis, or lateral ankle impingement is present. Stress lateral radiographs can be taken if lateral ankle instability is suspected (**Tables 1** and **2**).

CT is often used to evaluate for interval healing given the irregular anatomy of the calcaneus and joint arthrosis and to obtain a three-dimensional view through reconstruction views for surgical planning. In 1996 Stephens and Sanders[8] classified calcaneal malunions based on the CT scan and provided treatment recommendations based on a three-tier classification system. Type 1 malunion involves a lateral wall

Table 1
Complications from calcaneal fracture malunions

Diagnosis	Clinical Findings	Diagnostic Modalities
Hammertoe deformities	Hammertoe deformities	Radiographs reveal digital contractures Probable late complication of missed compartment syndrome
Peroneal impingement or subluxation/dislocation	Pain and edema posterolateral malleolus	Tenosynovitis, rupture, or subluxed on MRI
Cutaneous nerve injury or nerve entrapment	Severe poorly localized pain Sensory changes and paresthesias along the tibial or sural nerve	Positive electrophysiologic findings May warrant work-up for chronic pain syndrome by performing lumbar sympathetic blocks
Varus deformity of calcaneus	Hindfoot varus deformity in stance and with Coleman block, limited subtalar eversion, abnormal gait	Calcaneal varus deformity on hindfoot alignment views
Loss of calcaneal height	Anterior ankle joint pain and impingement Loss of push-off with ambulation Inability to fit in shoe wear	Loss of declination of the talus in relation to the floor
Widening of the calcaneus	Lateral ankle and subfibular impingement	Decreased calcaneal inclination angle Increased calcaneal width on calcaneal axial radiograph
Ankle arthritis	Ankle pain Aggravated walking uphill	Tibiotalar impingement, osteochondral defect, decrease in talar declination
Ankle instability	Ankle pain Instability reported Positive anterior drawer or talar tilt examination	Positive stress lateral radiographs Chronic lateral ankle ligament tear on MRI
Heel pain and exostosis	Chronic heel pain, aggravated with activity Fat pad atrophy	Prominent exostosis apparent on radiographs of the calcaneus Decreased height from floor to calcaneus on lateral foot radiograph

Table 2
Procedures for addressing calcaneal fracture malunions

Procedure	Rationale
Lateral wall exostosectomy	Decompresses lateral osseous impingement
Peroneal tendon repair	Repair of superior peroneal retinaculum or peroneal tendons
Sural neurolysis or resection	Nerve decompression or resection for nerve injury
Calcaneal osteotomy	Corrects malunion and residual deformity
Resection of tibia/talar exostosis	Corrects adaptive anterior ankle joint impingement
Lateral ligament repair or rerouting of the peroneal brevis	Prevents ankle instability
Subtalar bone block arthrodesis	Restores calcaneal height and corrects residual frontal plane deformities Addresses arthrosis of the subtalar joint Restores talocalcaneal angle
Triple arthrodesis	Addresses symptomatic subtalar and calcaneal cuboid arthrosis

exostosis, with or without partial subtalar arthrosis. Type 2 malunion involves a lateral wall exostosis with subtalar arthrosis involving the entire width of the subtalar joint. Type 3 malunion involves a lateral wall exostosis, subtalar arthrosis, and a varus malalignment of the calcaneal body.[8]

Before performing any calcaneal osteotomy to correct a residual deformity, deep hardware may need to be removed. A review of medical records or operative reports will assist the surgeon in acquiring the proper instrumentation needed for hardware removal. Calcaneal plates can be removed through alternative incisions such as those used for an osteotomy or subtalar joint fusion to possibly avoid wound healing complications. Small percutaneous incisions directly over the screws are used to remove the screws, and the plate is removed through the incision for the osteotomy or subtalar joint arthrodesis. At times, the extensile lateral incision ensures proper exposure for removal of the internal plate and screws.

SURGICAL OPTIONS FOR RESIDUAL CALCANEAL FRACTURE DEFORMITIES

This article discusses two of the most common deformities that are encountered and how they are successfully revised to further improve the patient's gait and functional abilities. The deformities are residual hindfoot varus and subtalar joint depression. At times, the surgeon will have to assess the patient on multiple occasions to determine the best suited procedures before performing revisional surgery. The following sections discuss the surgical options with calcaneal osteotomies and with subtalar joint distraction bone block arthrodesis for malunions without and with subtalar joint arthrosis, respectively.

Malunion Treated with Calcaneal Osteotomy

Joint salvage procedures are performed for malunions with minimal subtalar joint arthrosis. Calcaneal osteotomies have been reported to reorient the hindfoot alignment.[15–17] This method can be combined with arthrodesis in the presence of concomitant subtalar joint arthrosis.

Calcaneal varus deformities are best managed through a closing wedge osteotomy of the calcaneal tuberosity if a subtalar joint arthrodesis is not indicated. The osteotomy is performed through an oblique incision just posterior to peroneal tendons. The sural nerve is retracted and a periosteal incision made in the same path as the planned osteotomy. The lateral closing wedge osteotomy is then performed with a wide sagittal saw blade and fixated with either cannulated screws or staples. Often, a surgical dilemma arises when a calcaneal varus deformity is associated with a painful subtalar joint arthrosis. The surgeon often contemplates whether a calcaneal osteotomy is needed in conjunction with the subtalar joint arthrodesis. The rationale may be to correct the varus position through the subtalar joint level. Unfortunately, the varus deformity is a result of malreduction of the calcaneal tuberosity and medial wall of the calcaneus, and, unless it is corrected, residual varus deformity will occur despite trying to place the heel in a valgus position while performing the subtalar joint arthrodesis.

In addition, further lateral impingement can occur if correction of the varus deformity is performed by placing the subtalar joint into a valgus position to correct for a calcaneal varus deformity. Often, what occurs is a subtalar joint fusion with the lateral wall of the calcaneus against the distal tip of the fibula, impinging the peroneal tendons with the calcaneal tuberosity still in varus. If a subtalar joint arthrodesis is to be performed with a calcaneal osteotomy, it is the authors' preference to perform an oblique osteotomy across the healed primary fracture line. The main advantage of this procedure is that the same incision is used for both the osteotomy and joint arthrodesis, minimizing any potential soft tissue complications.

An oblique incision is centered over the sinus tarsi and is extended slightly posterior to offer exposure of the lateral wall of the calcaneus. This incision can be used for removal of a calcaneal plate when combined with small percutaneous incisions for removal of the screws. The extensor digitorum brevis is reflected distally, and soft tissue interposition across the sinus tarsi is excised. Identification of the posterior facet of the subtalar joint is then obtained using a curved osteotome. After the soft tissues between the talus and calcaneus are incised, a lamina spreader is placed into the sinus tarsi and distracted to expose the posterior facet of the subtalar joint. The remaining articular cartilage and subchondral plate of the talus and calcaneus are removed. It is important to try and maintain the normal contour of the joint. The primary fracture line is then identified and confirmed with a Steinman pin under fluoroscopy with a calcaneal axial view. Caution should be employed to place the Steinman pin posterior and inferior to the neurovascular bundle. It is not uncommon to see the primary fracture line partially united, in which case the osteotomy can be completed with a small curette or osteotome. If the primary fracture line is completely united, a wide osteotome is used to create the osteotomy using the placement of the Steinman pin as a guide.

The most difficult portion of the procedure is in positioning the calcaneal tuberosity. After the osteotomy is performed, a smooth lamina spreader is placed into the osteotomy and distracted to relax the soft tissues. A Schantz pin is then placed into the calcaneal tuberosity and used for positioning in combination with osteotomes as levers across the osteotomy and under the sustentacular fragment. After realignment is achieved, provisional fixation with Steinman pins across the osteotomy is performed. Small fragment screws are then used to fixate the osteotomy from lateral to medial aiming 15 to 20 degrees inferior. Screws located in this direction are placed directly across the osteotomy while still allowing an area for placement of a screw across the arthrodesis site. Typically, two screws are used to prevent rotation across the osteotomy. After the osteotomy is positioned, a 6.5- or 7.0-cannulated screw is placed from the posterior plantar aspect of the calcaneal tuberosity into the body of the talus crossing the posterior facet of the subtalar joint. Morcelized bone graft can then be placed across the subtalar joint, sinus tarsi, and the bone defect created on the lateral aspect from shifting of the tuberosity fragment.

The wounds are then closed in a layered fashion. A posterior splint is applied and later converted to a below-the-knee cast once edema subsides. The patient is kept strictly non–weight bearing, usually for 4 to 6 weeks for isolated osteotomy and 6 to 8 weeks for osteotomy and subtalar joint arthrodesis. A short leg walking cast is then applied for 4 weeks, followed by a walking boot for an additional 4 weeks. Physical therapy can be instituted to decrease edema, perform gait training, and improve range of motion of the subtalar joint (if an arthrodesis was not performed) and ankle joint.

Malunions Treated with Subtalar Joint Distraction Bone Block Arthrodesis

A subtalar joint distraction bone block arthrodesis is indicated when a subtalar joint arthrodesis needs to be performed but significant vertical collapse of the hindfoot is present.[18] In 1943 Gallie[19] described a technique of subastragalar arthrodesis in which a corticocancellous bone graft from the ipsilateral anteromedial tibia was placed across the subtalar joint from a posterolateral approach. This procedure was not recommended for feet with hindfoot varus deformities due to the fear of varus malunion. In 1988 Carr and colleagues[20] modified this approach by distracting the subtalar joint and placing tricortical structural intercalary bone blocks into the joint to maintain the correction. Because the operation as described was limited to a straight posterior incision, it was not possible to narrow the lateral wall, minimize the fibular impingement, release the calcaneocuboid joint, or reposition the subluxed and dislocated peroneal tendons. The main objective with this approach was restoration of the talocalcaneal relationship. By restoring talocalcaneal height, the long axis of the talus was made more vertical relative to the plane of support, relieving tibial impingement on the talar neck anteriorly and improving ankle dorsiflexion.

In 1993 Romash[17] described a reconstructive osteotomy of the calcaneus with subtalar joint arthrodesis. The Romash osteotomy recreated the primary fracture line and permitted repositioning of the tuberosity to narrow the heel, alleviate ankle impingement, and restore the height of the calcaneus. The fusion addressed symptoms of posttraumatic arthritis of the subtalar joint. The difference between the Romash osteotomy with subtalar joint fusion from the recommendations described previously is that it eliminated the need for cortical bone grafts for stability.[17] In 2005 Clare and colleagues[1] reported intermediate long-term results of their treatment protocol for calcaneal fracture malunions. For type 3 calcaneal fracture malunions, the following procedures were performed: a lateral wall exostosectomy, peroneal tenolysis, subtalar bone block arthrodesis, and a lateral closing wedge osteotomy of the calcaneus.[1]

Herein, the authors describe their preferred method of dealing with calcaneal malunions and concomitant subtalar joint arthrosis. When performing a subtalar joint distraction bone block arthrodesis, a vertical incision is preferred to prevent skin necrosis and wound healing complications. The extensile lateral incision can create significant tension of the horizontal limb after distraction of the subtalar joint and reconstitution of the calcaneal height. Nevertheless, some authorities report that the lateral extensile incision is reasonable because reconstructive surgery is performed when there is no acute edema or vascular compromise to the flap, and aggressive resection of the lateral wall will also decompress the flap.[1]

Hardware, if retained, can be removed from a vertical incision with the addition of small percutaneous incisions to remove the screws. If extensive hardware or broken hardware is present, requiring use of the extensile lateral incision, the distraction arthrodesis can be staged after removal of the hardware to prevent wound healing complications. The vertical incision is made along the posterior aspect of the ankle and extends to the inferior heel. The incision is typically 7 to 10 cm in length and positioned lateral and anterior to the Achilles tendon and posterior to the course of the sural nerve so that the nerve can be easily identified and retracted anteriorly.

Dissection begins with identification of the sural nerve and lesser saphenous vein in the proximal aspect of the incision. If the nerve after being inspected is severely scarred or if the patient displayed signs of painful sural neuritis preoperatively, the nerve is transected and buried into the peroneal muscle belly or through a small drill hole in the proximal fibula. The superior peroneal retinaculum is transected posterior to the peroneal tendons, exposing the peroneal tendon sheaths. The tendon sheaths of the peroneal tendons are maintained and retracted anteriorly with the sural nerve. Identification of the posterior aspect of the subtalar joint can be difficult, and dissection begins on the posterior aspect of the calcaneus until the joint is identified. The flexor hallucis longus tendon is visualized after the deep crural fascia is incised and retracted medially with large retractors. It is imperative not to violate the ankle joint because the talus is usually embedded into the body of the calcaneus. A half-inch curved osteotome is then used to mobilize and identify the posterior facet of the subtalar joint. After the joint is mobilized with an osteotome, a lamina spreader is placed to distract the joint. The remaining articular cartilage, soft tissue interposition, and subchondral plate are removed from the talus and calcaneus. All avascular and sclerotic bone must be resected for a successful union across the arthrodesis site. It is important to inspect the lateral wall of the calcaneus for subfibular impingement which is commonly encountered. An exostosectomy of the lateral wall of the calcaneus may be indicated if impingement persists.

Bone obtained from the exostectomy should be preserved in saline and later morcelized as supplement bone graft for the distraction arthrodesis and across any residual small defects. The alignment is viewed under C-arm fluoroscopy while the joint is distracted to determine the size of bone graft indicated to distract the joint. Normal declination of the talus needs to be confirmed while the joint is distracted with the lamina spreader before selecting the size of the graft. A structural allograft fashioned from a femoral head is used. The shape of the graft is trapezoidal, being slightly higher posteriorly and medially (correcting a varus deformity) or laterally (correcting a valgus deformity). Once the graft is fashioned, a smooth lamina spreader is placed into the joint under maximum tension, and the graft is tamped in. The graft and arthrodesis site are then stabilized with two 6.5 or 7.0 cannulated screws from the posteroinferior aspect of the calcaneus across the graft and into the body and neck of the talus (**Figs. 1** and **2**). Close attention to screw placement can also achieve correction at the talonavicular joint if placed precisely. The first screw is placed into the neck of the talus from the posteroinferior aspect of the calcaneal tuberosity. A short partially threaded screw when compressed leads to further declination of the talus and correction at the talonavicular joint. Alternatively, screws may be placed through a second incision from the superolateral talar shoulder, or from the dorsal aspect of the talar neck into the calcaneal body or anterior process of the calcaneus. The second screw is placed from the posteroinferior aspect of the calcaneal tuberosity into the body of the talus. A fully threaded screw can be placed if the graft has fractured upon insertion or if further collapse is a concern. Additional bone graft (harvested from the lateral calcaneal exostosectomy) and morcelized cancellous chips can be placed

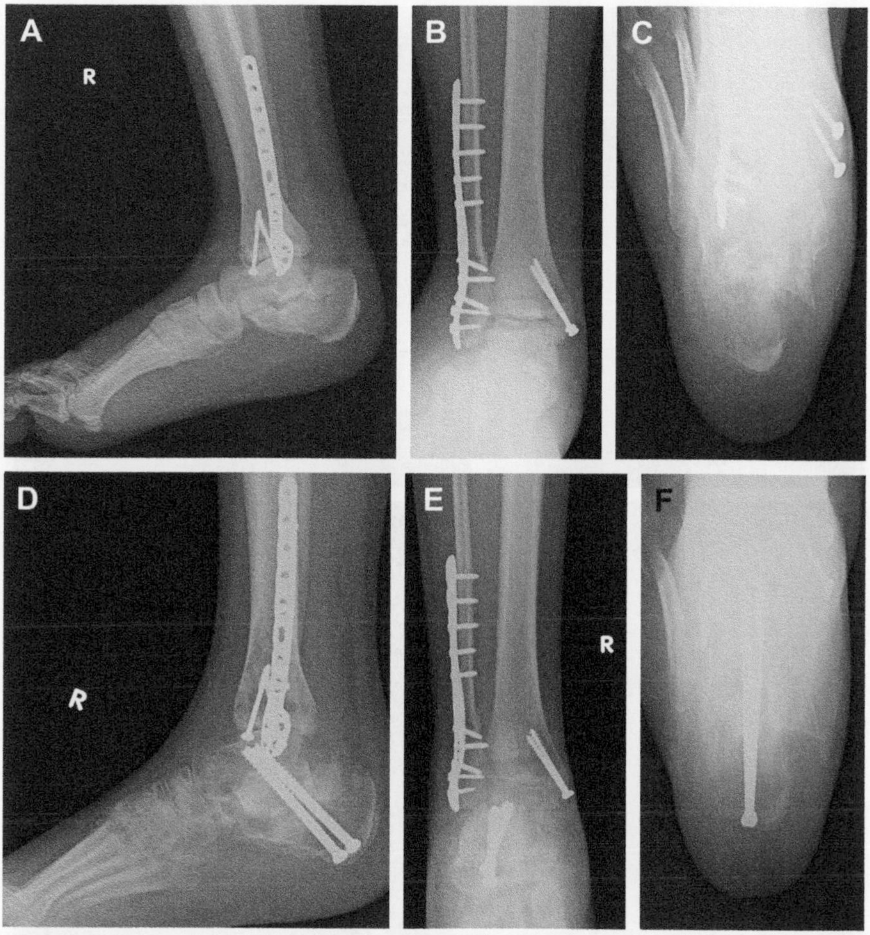

Fig. 1. Lateral ankle (*A*), anteroposterior ankle (*B*), and calcaneal axial (*C*) radiographic views showing a severe subtalar joint depression of the posterior facet. The patient sustained a grade 3 open ankle and calcaneal fracture. The surgery initially consisted of irrigation and debridement of the open wounds with open reduction and internal fixation of the ankle fracture. Further reconstruction was achieved by a bone block distraction arthrodesis of the subtalar joint. Note the declination of the talus and the correction of the anterior ankle joint impingement (*D–F*).

around the graft to augment the arthrodesis and to fill any small defects. If a varus or valgus deformity is present after insertion of the graft, the lateral or medial aspect of the calcaneus inferior to the graft can be tamped down to correct any residual deformity. All wounds are then closed in a layered fashion. A posterior splint is applied and is later converted into a cast when the edema subsides. The patient is kept strictly non–weight bearing for 8 to 10 weeks to prevent collapse of the graft. A short leg walking cast is then used for an additional 4 to 6 weeks, followed by a removable walking boot for 4 to 6 weeks. Physical therapy can assist with edema control, gait training, and ankle joint range of motion.

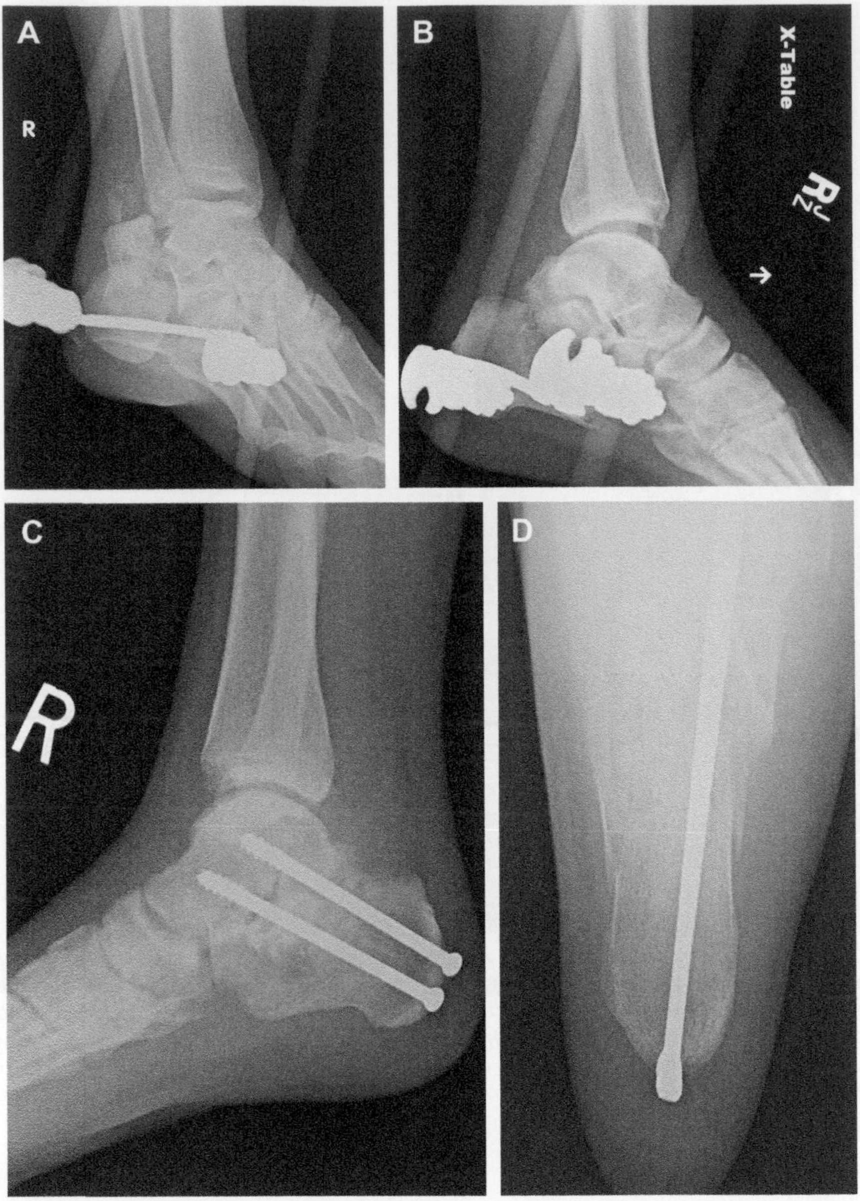

Fig. 2. Lateral radiographs (*A, B*) showing a pulverized grade 3 open calcaneal fracture after distraction with an external fixator. Note the displacement of the posterior facet and severe deformity. Revisional surgery was performed after the open fracture wound had healed and the patient displayed no clinical signs of infection. Surgery consisted of a calcaneal osteotomy across the healed primary fracture line, repositioning the calcaneal tuberosity, and performing a subtalar joint arthrodesis. Note the use of two 6.5-mm cannulated screws for fixation (*C, D*).

SUMMARY

Malunions of the calcaneus after operative intervention are debilitating for the patient and challenging for the treating physician. Calcaneal fractures are associated with a multitude of complications that can occur. A careful clinical and radiographic evaluation along with surgical techniques that are designed to reconstitute the normal anatomy of the calcaneus as it articulates with the remainder of the foot and ankle are paramount to decrease the patient's pain and improve gait and function. Realistic expectations and surgical goals have to be considered. In certain circumstances, pain can be decreased and function improved but rarely to preinjury levels.

REFERENCES

1. Clare MP, Lee WE, Sanders RW. Intermediate to long-term results of a treatment protocol for calcaneal fracture malunions. J Bone Joint Surg Am 2005;87(5): 963–73.
2. Cotton F, Henderson F. Results of fractures of the os calcis. Am J Orthop Surg 1916;14:290.
3. Levy LJ, Lipscomb CP, McDonald HC Jr, et al. Fractures of the os calcis: late functional results. Tex State J Med 1961;57:758–62.
4. Spranger M, Rabenseifner L. Late sequelae of calcaneal fractures. Z Orthop Ihre Grenzgeb 1975;113(4):686–8.
5. Zwipp H. Reconstructive surgery of malunited joint fractures of the foot. Orthopade 1990;19(6):409–15.
6. Myerson M, Quill GE Jr. Late complications of fractures of the calcaneus. J Bone Joint Surg Am 1993;75(3):331–41.
7. Wright DG, Sangeorzan BJ. Calcaneal fracture with peroneal impingement and tendon dysfunction. Foot Ankle Int 1996;17(10):650.
8. Stephens HM, Sanders R. Calcaneal malunions: results of a prognostic computed tomography classification system. Foot Ankle Int 1996;17(7):395–401.
9. Sangeorzan BJ. Salvage procedures for calcaneus fractures. Instr Course Lect 1997;46:339–46.
10. Zwipp H, Rammelt S. Posttraumatic deformity correction at the foot. Zentralbl Chir 2003;128(3):218–26.
11. Walter JH Jr, Rockett MS, Goss LR. Complications of intra-articular fractures of the calcaneus. J Am Podiatr Med Assoc 2004;94(4):382–8.
12. Buckley RE, Tough S. Displaced intra-articular calcaneal fractures. J Am Acad Orthop Surg 2004;12(3):172–8.
13. Zgonis T, Roukis TS, Polyzois VD. The use of Ilizarov technique and other types of external fixation for the treatment of intra-articular calcaneal fractures. Clin Podiatr Med Surg 2006;23(2):343–53.
14. Wang JH, Wu Y, Wang Y, et al. Treatment of calcaneal malunion fracture with isolated subtalar arthrodesis. Zhonghua Yi Xue Za Zhi 2007;87(47):3343–5.
15. Romash MM. Calcaneal fractures: three-dimensional treatment. Foot Ankle 1988; 8(4):180–97.
16. Romash MM. Fracture of the calcaneus: an unusual fracture pattern with subtalar joint interposition of the flexor hallucis longus. A report of two cases. Foot Ankle 1992;13(1):32–41.

17. Romash MM. Reconstructive osteotomy of the calcaneus with subtalar arthrodesis for malunited calcaneal fractures. Clin Orthop Relat Res 1993;(290):157–67.
18. Klaue K. The reorienting subtalar arthrodesis. Orthopade 2006;35(4):380–6.
19. Gallie W. Subastragalar arthrodesis in fractures of the os calcis. J Bone Joint Surg Am 1943;25:731–6.
20. Carr J, Hansen S, Benirschke S. Subtalar distraction bone block fusion for late complications of os calcis fractures. Foot Ankle 1988;9:81–6.

Talus Fractures: Surgical Principles

Shannon M. Rush, DPM, FACFAS*, Meagan Jennings, DPM, AACFAS,
Graham A. Hamilton, DPM, FACFAS

KEYWORDS

• Talus • Fracture • Open reduction • Foot • Ankle

Surgical treatment of talus fractures is challenging for even the most skilled foot and ankle surgeons. Complicated fracture patterns combined with joint dislocation of variable degrees requires accurate assessment, sound understanding of principles of fracture care, and broad command of internal fixation techniques needed for successful surgical care. Elimination of unnecessary soft tissue dissection, a low threshold for surgical reduction, and liberal use of malleolar osteotomy to expose body fractures and detailed attention to fracture reduction and joint alignment are critical to the success of surgical reconstruction.

Descriptions of talus fractures are well documented[1–8] with little remaining to be said with regard to fracture pattern and classification schemes. Complications, such as infection, malunion, posttraumatic arthritis, osteonecrosis, and talar collapse, have been well documented and shown to be frequent complications of talus fractures.[7–12]

The vascular supply to the talus is robust receiving branches from all the vessels that supply distal runoff to the foot. Several studies have documented the extensive extraosseous and intraosseous blood supply to the talus.[13–17] Despite the rich circulation to the talus the vessels are easily compromised with injury of the talus by fracture and joint dislocation. Restoration of the extraosseous blood supply can only occur with accurate restoration of joint alignment. Restoring the intraosseous anastomoses, which are necessary for fracture healing and revascularization of the talar body, relies on anatomic fracture reduction and rigid internal fixation.

The most clinically significant complication after talar neck fracture is avascular necrosis (AVN) with collapse of the talar body. The incidence of radiographic AVN after talar neck fractures has been previously well documented.[7,8,18,19] More recently, MRI studies have shown the incidence of AVN to be higher with more accurate diagnostic imaging.[18,19] Thordarson and colleagues[18] were able to demonstrate radiographic evidence of AVN did not correlate with MRI findings except in cases in which greater than 50% of the talar body had AVN. Talar collapse, however, did not necessarily correlate with amount of AVN in the talar body. Vallier and colleagues[9] found AVN with collapse in

Department of Podiatric Surgery, Palo Alto Foundation Medical Foundation, Camino Division, 701 East El Camino Real, Mountain View, CA 94040, USA
* Corresponding author.
E-mail address: rushdoc@gmail.com (S.M. Rush).

Clin Podiatr Med Surg 26 (2009) 91–103
doi:10.1016/j.cpm.2008.09.007
podiatric.theclinics.com

31% of displaced talar neck fractures. In addition, there was no correlation between time to surgical reduction and development of AVN. AVN was more common in injures with medial neck comminution and open injuries signifying a higher energy injury pattern.[9]

Surgical care of talar body fractures is appropriately included in the same discussion of talar neck fractures. Fractures of the talar body are even more rare than talar neck fractures and are generally believed to be caused by high-energy axial loading of the tibiotalar joint. Posttraumatic arthritis, AVN, and malunion are common consequences of talar body fractures.[20–25] Vallier and colleagues[11] showed that 50% of body fractures that developed AVN eventually collapsed. By the nature of the injury, body fractures involve more of the articular surface of the tibiotalar joint and subtalar joint. Inokuchi and coworkers[20] suggested a consistent way to differentiate neck and body fractures based on the involvement of the subtalar joint, which may be valid for research purposes but does not have significant influence on surgical decision making. Surgical approaches and exposure of talar body fractures is difficult given the confines of the ankle joint and the medial and lateral malleoli.

Titanium internal fixation which causes less ferromagnetic interference with postreduction magnetic resonance scanning is generally recommended for surgical care (**Fig. 1**).[18] Less image distortion of the talar body allows for accurate assessment of avascular changes in the talar body. To date no studies have shown improved outcomes with titanium with respect to AVN or fracture healing. Often mini or small fragment plates can be used in addition to screws with the added disadvantage of soft tissue dissection from the body and neck of the talus.

SURGICAL TREATMENT OF TALAR NECK FRACTURES

Indications for open reduction and internal fixation should be liberal. The consequence of fracture malunion and subtalar varus will often lead to deformity and stiffness which requires early secondary reconstruction.[10] Grade 1 injuries without displacement should refer only to those fractures which have no displacement of the neck fracture. CT scanning accurately assesses the absence of neck fracture

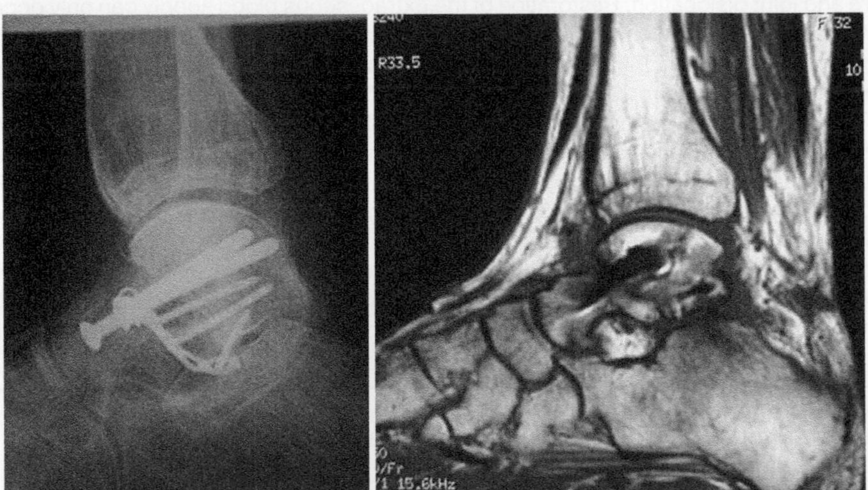

Fig. 1. Postreduction MRI of talus fracture with titanium fixation. There is a distinct signal void over the internal screws but little distortion of the remainder of the talar body. The degree of avascular necrosis can be assessed in the talar body.

displacement. Varus malalignment in the subtalar joint can be evaluated with plain radiographs of the foot demonstrated by a reduction in the talocalcaneal angle and increased coverage of the talar head (**Fig. 2**). Injuries meeting these criteria (ie, no displacement and no varus malalignment of the subtalar joint) are truly nondisplaced and usually require 6 weeks of immobilization for fracture healing. There is some controversy, however, surrounding the minimally displaced neck fracture with subtle varus rotational malalignment of the subtalar joint. In most circumstances the authors believe these injuries should undergo open reduction and internal fixation. Fracture stabilization allows early rehabilitation which minimizes stiffness in the hindfoot. Radiographs taken after casting should assess the talometatarsal axis and the position of the lateral process of the talus to the floor of the sinus tarsi.

Higher grades of injury almost exclusively require open reduction and internal fixation even in cases in which the closed reduction achieved reduction of the fracture. The dislocated talar body often is locked posterior to the subtalar facet in Grade 2 injuries and the posterior malleolus in Grade 3 injuries. Immediate closed reduction should always be attempted in the emergency department. After conscious sedation is administered, the knee is flexed to relax the gastrocnemius muscle. Distal traction and posterior manual pressure is applied to the dislocated talar body in Kagers triangle. A reasonable closed reduction can usually be achieved. Once relocated the ankle is splinted in slight plantarflexion to prevent recurrent posterior dislocation (**Fig. 3**).

Infrequently, the dislocated talar body becomes locked behind the posterior malleolus and closed reduction is unsuccessful. Urgent surgical reduction is necessary for these injuries. A femoral distractor applied to the medial side of ankle with a half pin in the tibia and one in the calcaneus is used to create separation between the calcaneus and posterior malleolus (**Fig. 4**). An additional posterior approach to reduce the

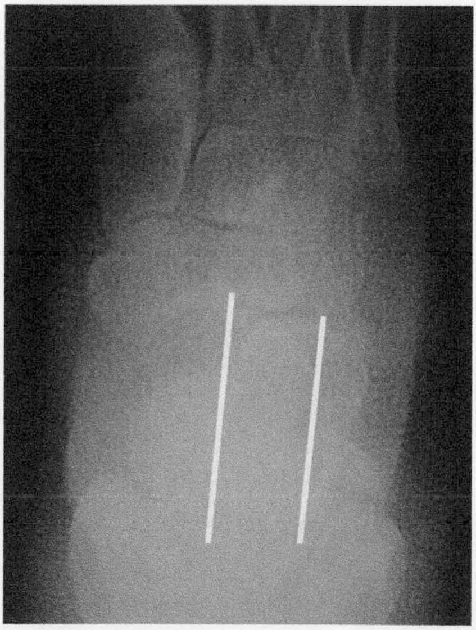

Fig. 2. Anteroposterior view of a nondisplaced talar neck fracture with varus hind foot alignment seen with loss of the talometatarsal axis and covering of the talar head. This subtle radiographic finding is suggestive of "varus" or external rotation malalignment of the subtalar joint.

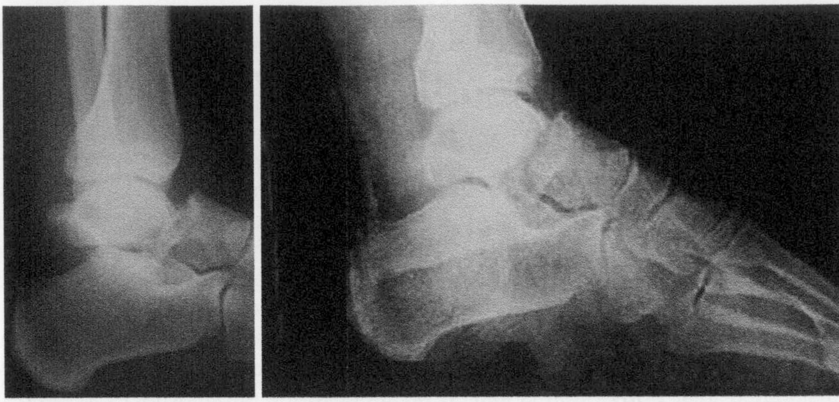

Fig. 3. Talar neck fracture after closed reduction and splinting. The ankle is held in slight plantarflexion to keep the talar body from dislocation.

talar body is not necessary. After appropriate distraction is applied a simple medial arthrotomy exposes the joint and dislocated talar body. Reduction of the body into the mortise is easily achieved. Alternatively, a Steinman pin can be placed through the Achilles tendon to aid in the reduction of the talar body.

The ideal surgical approach allows for direct and accurate exposure of the fracture allowing visualization of the anterior ankle joint. In addition, the surgical approach should allow for accurate placement of internal fixation. The authors favor the medial utility approach advocated by Sigvard T. Hansen, MD.[26] The incision is centered over the midline of the medial column and can be extended distally to the first metatarsophalangeal joint and posteriorly to the anterior border of the Achilles tendon for

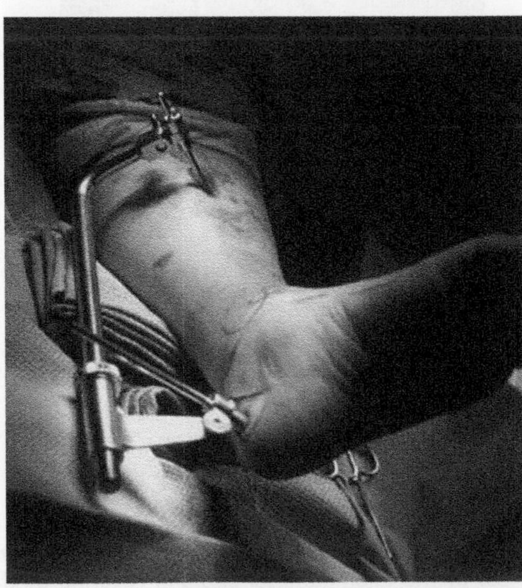

Fig. 4. Femoral distractor placed with one pin in the calcaneal tuberosity and one in the tibia aids in restoring separation between the calcaneus and tibia in an irreducible Grade 3 injury.

exposure of the posterior ankle and talus if necessary (**Fig. 5**). By design the incision is between the inner nervous planes and avoids most important neurovascular structures. Care should be taken to avoid unnecessary dissection of the soft tissue from the talar neck. Often the transverse fracture of the neck is posterior to the ankle capsule and a simple linear arthrotomy allows for visualization across the entire ankle, making reflection of the soft tissue of the talar neck unnecessary. For simple fracture patterns without medial comminution or bone loss a single medial approach is all that is necessary for accurate fracture reduction. A linear arthrotomy of the talonavicular joint and medial capsular reflection allows for exposure of the medial articular surface of the talar head (**Fig. 6**). Screws placed through the medial marginal articular surface are closer to perpendicular to the fracture and are countersunk beneath the articular surface. Occasionally, the navicular tuberosity is enlarged and a detriment to axial screw placement. A trough can be made in the navicular tuberosity with a power burr, which allows for better axial placement of screws. In the absence of medial neck comminution the interdigitation of the fracture with reduction affords excellent stability, and interfragmentary compression is recommended. When comminution of the medial neck is present or there is significant bone loss interfragmentary compression is generally not recommended because shortening of the medial neck occurs and varus malunion results (**Fig. 7**). There are two ways to assess whether proper length and alignment has been restored to the talar neck. The Canale view[8] is a modified oblique view of the foot to assess the length of the medial neck. Additionally, the talometarsal axis is assessed for residual malalignment (**Fig. 8**).

In cases of medial neck comminution with significant bone loss a medially placed plate and supplemental bone grafting in indicated.[27] The authors use distal tibial bone graft, which is harvested from the distal medial tibial crest (**Fig. 9**). This bicortical graft can be hand milled to fill any defect in the medial neck. The graft can then be secured with a medial bridge plate. Chateau and colleagues[27] showed in a small series of 23 comminuted neck fractures medial plating was effective and gave similar short-term results compared with screw fixation. An alternative to medial cortical bone graft and plating is initial reduction and fixation of the lateral side of the neck fracture first. Lateral neck comminution is less common, and with anatomic reduction of the lateral neck fracture with interfragmentary compression the length of the medial neck is restored. Positional screw fixation on the medial side adds stability.

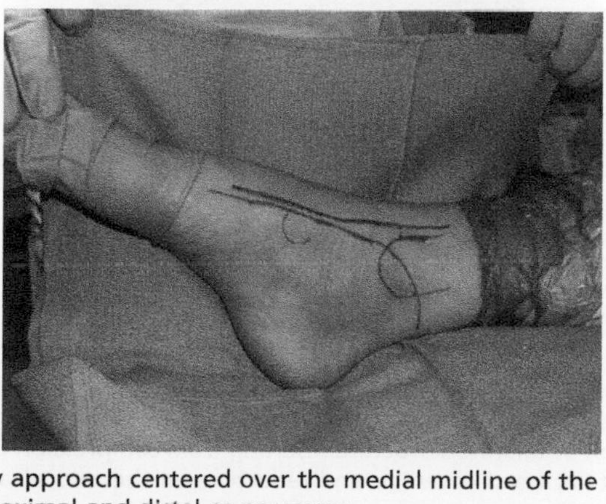

Fig. 5. Medial utility approach centered over the medial midline of the medial column and can be extended proximal and distal as necessary.

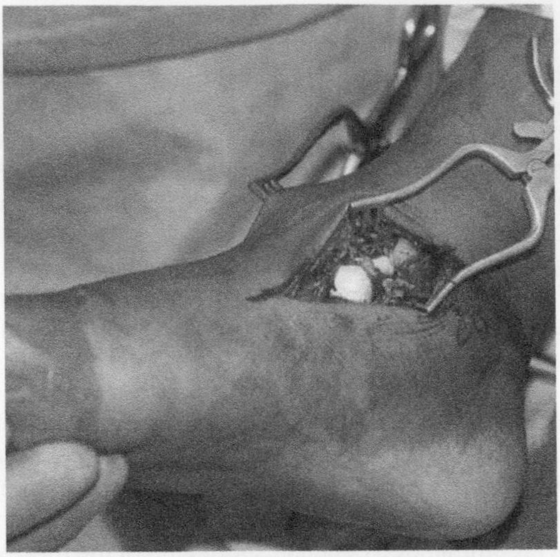

Fig. 6. Medial exposure of talar neck with linear arthrotomy of ankle and talonavicular joint. The fracture can be visualized inside the ankle capsule. The soft tissue is not dissected from the dorsal talar neck. The medial articular surface of the talar head is exposed for placement of fixation.

The anterolateral approach is necessary for fractures in which there is significant comminution of the medial neck with bone loss or fracture fragments involving the lateral talar neck or lateral process, which require open reduction internal fixation or debridement (**Fig. 10**). The anterolateral approach is made lateral and parallel to the extensor digitorum longus. The extensor digitorum brevis muscle belly is divided or

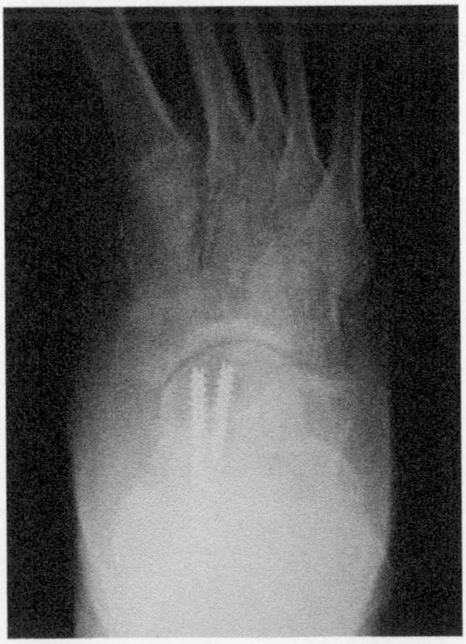

Fig. 7. Varus malunion of talar neck fracture resulting from compression of medial neck comminution. Increase talar head coverage and reduction on the talocalcaneal angle suggest varus malunion.

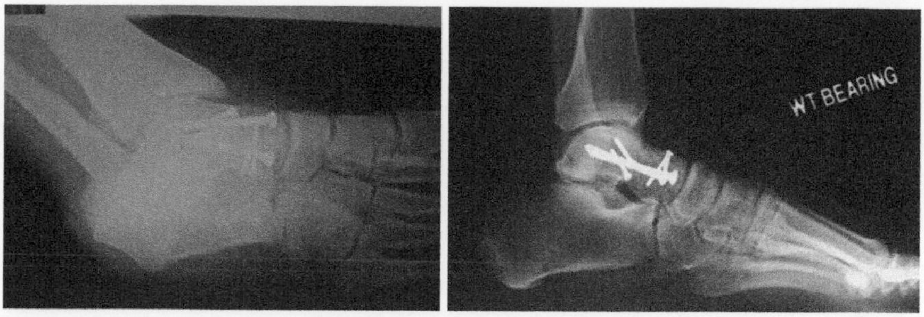

Fig. 8. Radiographic assessment of talar neck fracture after open reduction internal fixation. The Canale view and talometatarsal axis are additional indicators of proper reduction.

reflected laterally to allow for accurate and wide visualization of the lateral neck and lateral talonavicular joint. Dissection can be carried laterally over the body and lateral process to reduce lateral process fracture and debride bone debris in the sinus tarsi. Dissection into the sinus tarsi or beneath the talar neck should be avoided to minimize additional disruption of the tenuous blood supply.

Reduction of subtalar joint subluxation is often overlooked after fracture reduction and often leads to varus malalignment and postreduction stiffness. Subtle posterior translation and external rotation malalignment occasionally persists after fracture reduction. The best way to assess this is a lateral projection of the foot with the forefoot loaded. The author recommends using intraoperative radiographs verifying the reduction of the lateral process of the talus reduced to the floor of the sinus tarsi with ankle in dorsiflexion after fracture reduction. If the subtalar joint cannot be anatomically reduced a retrograde Steinman pin can be used to stabilize the subtalar joint while the ligamentous complex heals (**Fig. 11**).

The posterior approach for stabilization of talar neck fractures has been advocated,[28–31] although there are several disadvantages to this technique. Advocates of this technique cite that is a more stable fixation construct.[29] Placement of screws from the posterior aspect of the talus is technically difficult and positioning can be difficult. Additionally, more dissection is needed over the posterior talar body further compromising the tenuous blood supply. Damage to the flexor hallucis longus tendon, posterior ankle joint impingement on the screw heads, placement into the sinus tarsi, or violation of the subtalar joint with seating of the screws are all potential complications of posterior screw placement. In addition, as the screws are placed through the talar neck one must pay close attention to the oblique view of the neck intraoperatively to ensure that the screws do not traverse the sinus tarsi (**Fig. 12**).

SURGICAL TREATMENT OF TALAR BODY FRACTURES

The most significant obstacle to proper reduction of talar body fracture is adequate exposure. Without adequate exposure of the trochlear surface of the talus, reduction and fixation cannot be accomplished. Sneppen and Buhl[24] described fractures of the body generally with five separate categories: (1) transchondral fractures; (2) osteochondral fractures; (3) body fractures (coronal, sagittal, or horizontal shear fractures); (4) process fractures (posterior and lateral); and (5) crush fractures of the whole body. Isolated process fractures and osteochondral fractures can be treated with a direct surgical exposure and internal fixation or arthroscopic reduction. Complex fractures

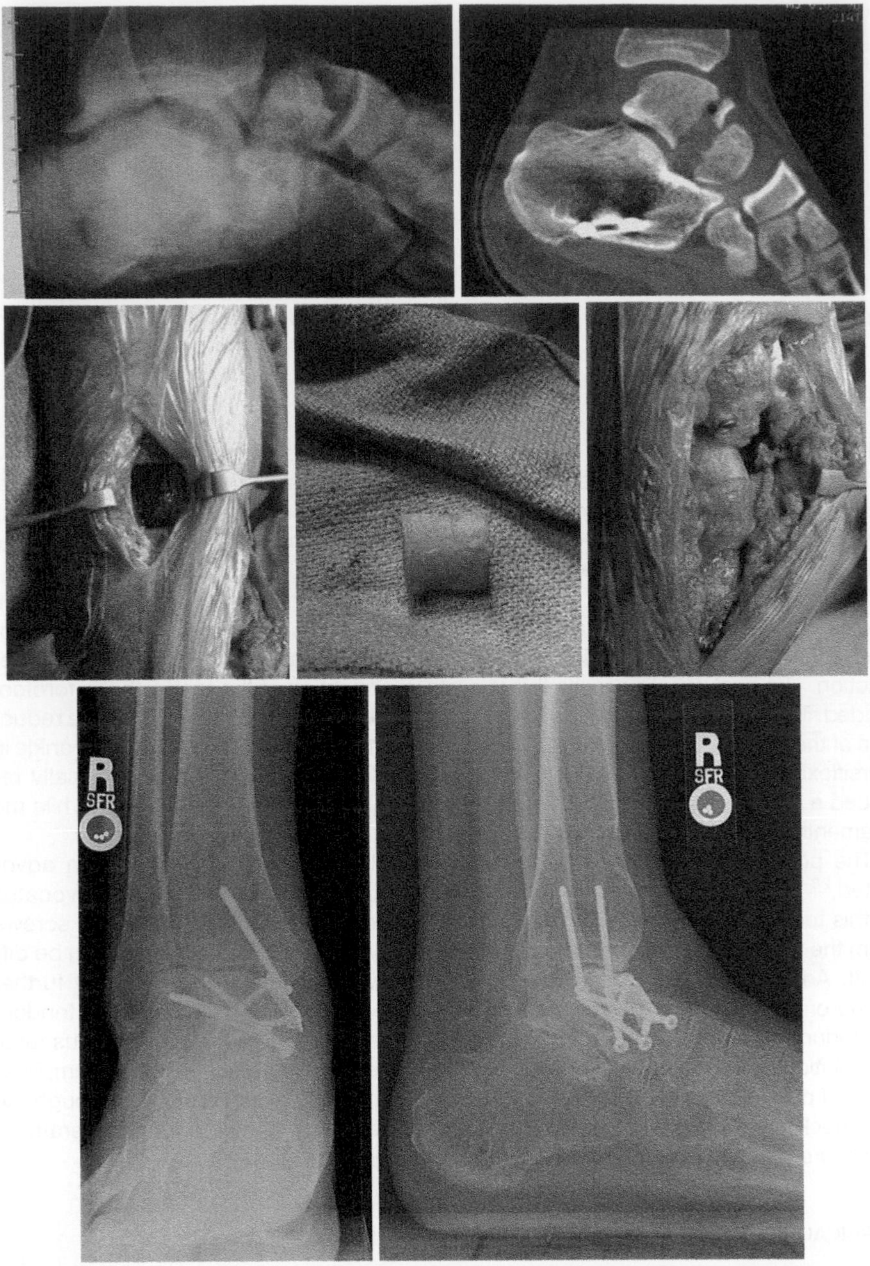

Fig. 9. Grade 4 open neck fracture with significant bone loss of the neck. A corticocancellous graft harvested from the distal medial tibia is hand milled to reconstruct the talar neck. The neck fracture is stabilized with positional screws and a two-hole plate. One year follow up after open reduction. Avascular necrosis without collapse developed in this patient.

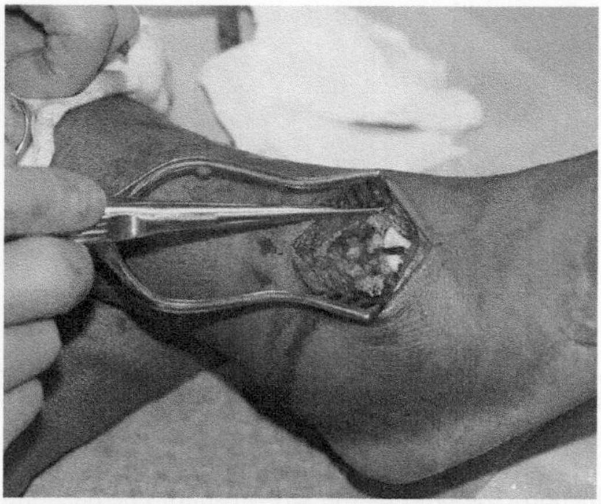

Fig. 10. Anterolateral approach. The incision is made lateral and parallel to the extensor digitorum longus tendon. The inferior extensor retinaculum is divided and the extensor digitorum brevis muscle belly can be split or reflected laterally to allow for accurate and wide visualization of the lateral neck and lateral talonavicular joint.

of the talar body require visualization of the trochlear surface of the talus for anatomic reduction. Direct exposure can be accomplished with medial or lateral malleolar osteotomy. Osteotomy allows for direct exposure of the articular surface and eliminates the need for soft tissue dissection around the ankle joint. A direct transosseous approach is often made possible through an existing medial malleolar fracture.

Medial malleolar osteotomy is the most common osteotomy performed for reduction of complex talar body fractures.[32] The medial malleolus is exposed from a direct medial incision. Careful attention to make the osteotomy enter the ankle joint just lateral to the axilla of the ankle joint ensures the entire trochlear surface of the joint can be visualized. The screw holes for reduction of the malleolus are predrilled to facilitate anatomic reduction of the malleolus after talar reduction (**Fig. 13**). The medial malleolus is reflected inferior to expose the talar body. The area of the talus just above

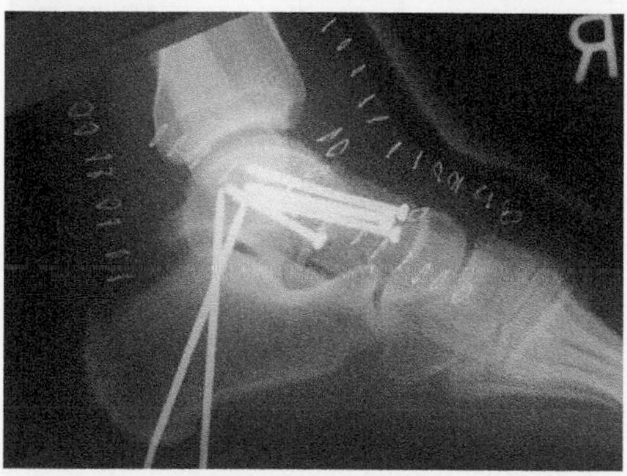

Fig. 11. Retrograde pinning of the subtalar joint. The lateral process of the talus is reduced to the floor of the sinus tarsi and pinned ensuring proper reduction of the subtalar joint.

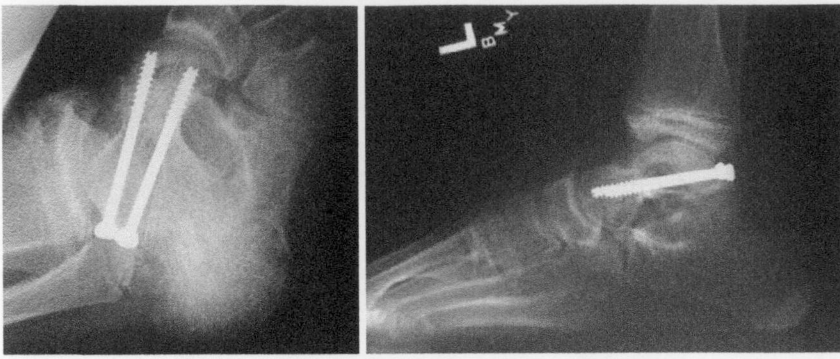

Fig. 12. Posterior screw placement. Oblique views of the hindfoot are needed to ensure the placement of the lateral screw does not violate the sinus tarsi, which is a common mistake leading to poor reduction. The land of the screw cannot encroach into the subtalar joint when seating the screw. Notice the prominence of the screw heads with plantarlexion of the ankle joint.

the deep deltoid ligament is often a good area for screw placement in difficult fracture patterns of the talar body. The screws can be placed in a subarticular fashion and buried in the subchondral bone to ensure no impingement with ankle motion occurs.

The fibular door osteotomy[28] described by Hansen is valuable for complex fractures of the lateral body of the talus. The primary indication for fibular osteotomy is a comminuted lateral talar body fracture involving both the lateral plafond and the lateral talar process. Often these fractures are difficult to expose. The fibular osteotomy is made through a straight lateral incision. Intraoperative imaging ensures the transverse osteotomy is made into the syndesmotic recess. A periosteal sleeve, which includes the anterotalofibular ligament and calcaneofibular ligament, is reflected in one soft

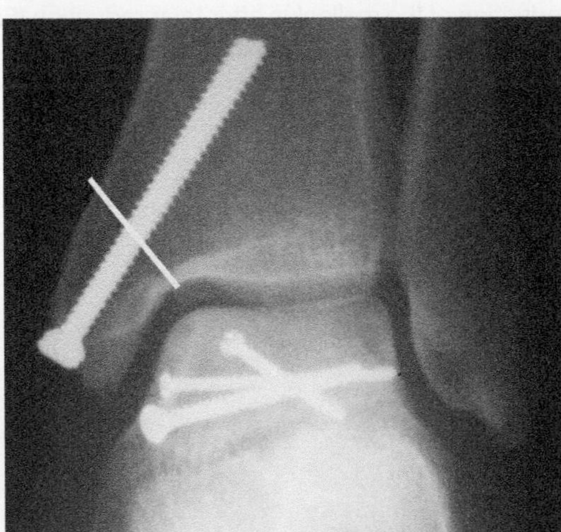

Fig. 13. Medial malleolar osteotomy. Using fluoroscopic guidance to ensure the osteotomy is made just lateral to the axilla of the tibia ensures visualization of the trochlear surface of the talus.

tissue envelope for later repair. The fibula is then opened like a "door" on the posterior peroneal retinacular and ligamentous "hinge" (**Fig. 14**). The exposure allows for complete visualization of the lateral talus and trochlear surface without excessive soft tissue dissection into the sinus tarsi. Fixation of the fibular osteotomy can be done in a number of ways based on surgeon preference.

Fractures of the talus present significant surgical hurdles for the foot and ankle surgeon. There is no dogmatic way to approach all fractures and surgical algorithms are inadequate to include all variations of the injury. Even with accurate and appropriate surgical care morbidity is common. Sanders and colleagues[33] showed the need for secondary reconstructive surgery in 1 year was 24% and increased to 48% at 10 years. Additionally, varus malalignment led to more pain and lower functional outcome scores when compared with patients in which alignment was evaluated as normal. In contrast, patients who avoided complications, such as AVN and varus malalignment, scored significantly better in functional outcomes. The most common reason for secondary surgery was subtalar arthritis.[33]

With any complex fracture the basic tenets of fracture care apply and talus fractures are no exception. Physical examination, reduction of dislocations, splinting, and medical observation of the patient are the foundation for surgical care. Assessment of the soft tissue envelope should guide the foot and ankle surgeon to the appropriate time for fracture reduction. Each fracture should be assessed individually and often CT scanning is a valuable tool for surgical planning. The surgical plan should include a direct well-planned surgical exposure to the fracture and allow for direct reduction and placement of fixation, avoidance of soft tissue complications by allowing sufficient time for soft tissue edema to subside, eliminating unnecessary soft tissue dissection, anatomic fracture reduction, and joint realignment.

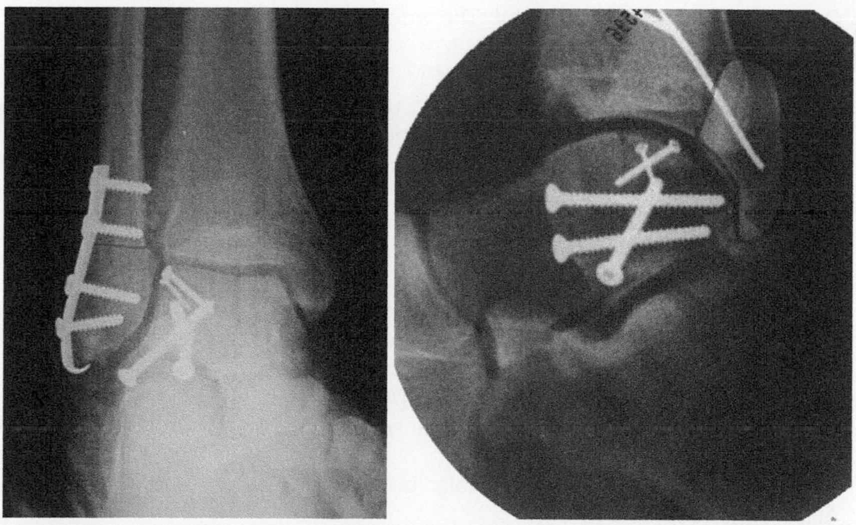

Fig. 14. Fibular door osteotomy. Transverse osteotomy made at the level of the syndesmotic recess. The soft tissue and ligamentous attachments are reflected as a single sleeve distally and are easily reattached with suture and drill holes made into the fibula after reduction of the talus and fixation of the osteotomy. The fibula is rotated posterior on the soft tissue hinge.

REFERENCES

1. Coltart W. Aviator's astragalus. J Bone Joint Surg Br 1952;34:545–66.
2. Syme J. Contributions to the pathology and practice of surgery. Edinburgh (UK): Sutherland and Knox; 1848.
3. Stealy J. Fractures of the astragalus. Surg Gynecol Obstet 1909;8:36.
4. Anderson HG. The medical and surgical aspects of aviation. London: Oxford Medical Publications; 1919.
5. Pennal GF. Fractures of the talus. Clin Orthop 1963;30:53–63.
6. Kleiger B. Fractures of the talus. J Bone Joint Surg Am 1948;30:735–44.
7. Hawkins LG. Fractures of the neck of the talus. J Bone Joint Surg Am 1970;52: 991–1002.
8. Canale ST, Kelly FB Jr. Fractures of the neck of the talus: long-term evaluation of seventy-one cases. J Bone Joint Surg Am 1978;60:143–56.
9. Vallier HA, Nork SE, Barei DP, et al. Talar neck fractures: results and outcomes. J Bone Joint Surg Am 2004;86:1616–24.
10. Daniels TR, Smith JW, Ross TI. Varus malalignment of the talar neck: its effect on the position of the foot and on subtalar motion. J Bone Joint Surg Am 1996;78: 1559–67.
11. Vallier HA, Nork SE, Barei DP, et al. Surgical treatment of talar body fractures. J Bone Joint Surg Am 2003;85:1716–24.
12. Szyszkowitz R, Reschauer R, Seggl W. Eighty-five talus fractures treated by ORIF with five to eight years of follow-up study of 69 patients. Clin Orthop 1985;199: 97–107.
13. Kelly PJ, Sullivan CR. Blood supply of the talus. Clin Orthop 1963;30:37–44.
14. Peterson L, Goldie I, Lindell D. The arterial supply of the talus. Acta Orthop Scand 1974;45:260–70.
15. Mulfinger GL, Trueta J. The blood supply of the talus. J Bone Joint Surg Br 1970; 52:160–7.
16. Gelberman RH, Mortensen WW. The arterial anatomy of the talus. Foot Ankle 1983;4:64–72.
17. Haliburton RS, Kelly PJ, Peterson LFA. The extra-osseous and intra-osseous blood supply of the talus. J Bone Joint Surg Am 1958;40:1115–20.
18. Thordarson DB, Triffon MJ, Terk MR. Magnetic resonance imaging to detect avascular necrosis after open reduction and internal fixation of talar neck fractures. Foot Ankle Int 1996;17:742–7.
19. Henderson RC. Posttraumatic necrosis of the talus: the Hawkins sign versus magnetic resonance imaging. J Orthop Trauma 1991;5:96–9.
20. Inokuchi S, Ogawa K, Usami N. Classification of fractures of the talus: clear differentiation between neck and body fractures. Foot Ankle Int 1996;17:748–50.
21. Trillat A, Bousquet G, Lapeyre B. [Displaced fractures of the neck or of the body of the talus: value of screwing by posterior surgical approach]. Rev Chir Orthop Reparatrice Appar Mot 1970;56:529–36 [Article in French].
22. Frawley PA, Hart JA, Young DA. Treatment outcome of major fractures of the talus. Foot Ankle Int 1995;16:339–45.
23. Faraj AA, Watters AT. Combined talar body and tibial plafond fracture. J Foot Ankle Surg 1999;38:888–91.
24. Sneppen O, Buhl O. Fracture of the talus: a study of its genesis and morphology based upon cases with associated ankle fracture. Acta Orthop Scand 1974;45: 307–20.

25. Saltzman CL, Marsh JL, Tearse DS. Treatment of displaced talus fractures: an arthroscopically assisted approach. Foot Ankle Int 1994;15:630–3.
26. Hansen ST Jr. Functional reconstruction of the foot and ankle. p. 544. Hagerstown: Lippincott Williams & Wilkins; 2000.
27. Chateau PB, Brokaw DS, Jelen BA, et al. Plate fixation of talar neck fractures: preliminary review of a new technique in twenty-three patients. J Orthop Trauma 2002;16(4):213–9.
28. Ebraheim NA, Mekhail AO, Salpietro BJ, et al. Talar neck fractures: anatomic considerations for posterior screw application. Foot Ankle Int 1996;17:541–7.
29. Lemaire RG, Bustin W. Screw fixation of fractures of the neck of the talus using a posterior approach. J Trauma 1980;20:669–73.
30. Mayo K. Fractures of the talus: principles of management and techniques of treatment. Tech Orthop 1987;2:42–54.
31. Swanson TV, Bray TJ, Holmes GB Jr. Fractures of the talar neck: a mechanical study of fixation. J Bone Joint Surg Am 1992;74:544–51.
32. Ziran BH, Abidi NA, Scheel MJ. Medial malleolar osteotomy for exposure of complex talar body fractures. J Orthop Trauma 2001;15(7):513–8.
33. Sanders DW, Busam M, Hattwick E, et al. functional outcomes after talar neck fractures. J Orthop Trauma 2004;18(5):265–70.

Management of Complications of Open Reduction and Internal Fixation of Ankle Fractures

Alan Ng, DPM, FACFAS*, Esther S. Barnes, DPM

KEYWORDS

• Ankle fracture complications • Nonunion
• Malunion • Open reduction

The outcome of the reduction of a displaced ankle fracture depends on the severity of the injury,[1] the degree of talar displacement before reduction, the type of fracture, and the presence of deltoid ligament rupture as quantified by an increase in the width of the medial clear space.[2–4] Age, sex, and completeness of restoration of the distal tibiofibular syndesmosis are other factors that have been shown to affect the final clinical result.[2,3] Adequate reduction is critical, with reduction of the lateral malleolus to restore normal length and produce correct alignment of the talus within the mortise being most important.[5]

The management of complications resulting from the open reduction and internal fixation (ORIF) of ankle fractures is discussed in detail. The initial radiographic findings of the most common postsurgical complications of ankle fracture reduction are briefly discussed, namely lateral, medial, and posterior malleolar malunion or nonunion, syndesmotic widening, degenerative changes, and septic arthritis with or without concomitant osteomyelitis. Emphasis is placed on the management of these complications, with a review of the treatment options proposed in the literature, a detailed discussion of the authors' recommendations, and an inclusion of case presentations.

RADIOGRAPHIC EVALUATION

As proposed by Weber[6] in 1981, the normal ankle joint as seen with the 20° internally rotated anteroposterior view, or "mortise view," shows the following three

Highlands - Presbyterian/St. Luke's Podiatric Medicine and Surgery Residency Program, Denver, CO, USA
* Corresponding author. 8101 E. Lowry Boulevard, #230, Denver, CO 80230, USA.
E-mail address: ang@advancedortho.org (A. Ng).

Clin Podiatr Med Surg 26 (2009) 105–125
doi:10.1016/j.cpm.2008.09.008
podiatric.theclinics.com
0891-8422/08/$ – see front matter

characteristics: (1) a perfectly parallel and equidistant joint space, (2) a Shenton's line of the ankle in which a medial fibular spike, pointing to the level of the tibial subchondral bone, is noted while following the contour of the tibia over the syndesmotic space of the fibula, and (3) an unbroken curve between the lateral talar articular surface and recess of distal fibula where the peroneal tendons lie. In contrast to these normal findings, the mortise view of the "sprung mortise" shows the following: (1) a joint space that is no longer strictly parallel, particularly on the medial side where there is widening proportional to the degree of lateral shift of the talus, (2) a broken Shenton line of the ankle, with the small spike of the fibula lying more proximal as a result of shortening, and (3) a broken curve between the lateral part of the talar articular surface and the recess of the distal fibula as a result of fibular shortening.[6,7]

The medial clear space is perhaps the most widely used measurement of reduction. Less than a 1-mm space or more than a 4-mm space is correlated with a poor outcome.[8,9] The talocrural angle, which allows one to judge the length of the fibular reduction compared with the medial malleolus, is defined by a line drawn perpendicular to the tibial articular surface and a line connecting the distal aspects of the medial and lateral malleoli. Less than 2° difference from the contralateral ankle was deemed acceptable by Sarkisian and Cody,[10] who proposed the angle in 1976. Talar tilt has also been used by Offierski and colleagues[11] to assess proper reduction of the fibula. Lines are drawn along the surfaces of the talar dome and tibial plafond. In the normal and adequately reduced ankle these lines are parallel. Failure to correct this tilt to 1° or less was considered to be poor reduction.

The fibular malunions can be classified radiographically as either occult or overt malunions as defined by Yablon and Leach[12] in 1989. An *occult* malunion is one in which the talus remains in its normal position but the lateral malleolus shows residual displacement characterized by external rotation and shortening, whereas with an *overt* malunion, the talus is displaced in addition to the changes noted with the fibula. It is more difficult to diagnose an occult malunion because the talus appears to be in normal position. The use of CT scans may be recommended for cases in which lateral radiographs fail to show a malunion of the lateral malleolus but a high clinical suspicion is present.[12,13]

Radiographic evaluation of nonunions consists of determining whether the nonunion is hypertrophic or hypotrophic. Hypertrophic nonunions are characterized by significant bone production at the nonunion site, whereas hypotrophic, atrophic, or avascular nonunions demonstrate little evidence of bone production radiographically.[14,15] Further clarification of the type of nonunion can be delineated by bone scintigraphy or CT evaluation.

A lax syndesmotic ligament often presents itself radiographically as an enlarged medial clear space, increased to 2 to 3 mm, or a slight talar tilt.[16,17] Other radiographic criteria have been developed to diagnose the syndesmotic reduction more accurately.[18,19] The syndesmotic width is defined as the distance between the tibial incisura and the medial border of the fibula 1 cm proximal to the tibial joint surface. Another syndesmotic measurement involves the tibiofibular overlap from the fibular medial border to the lateral border of the anterior tibial prominence with less than 10 mm being abnormal.[8]

Radiographic signs of osteomyelitis include periostitis, soft tissue swelling, and rarefaction initially, followed by well-defined lytic lesions in bone with a dense sclerotic rim, namely Brodie abscesses.[20–23] Chronic osteomyelitis is characterized radiographically by bone lysis, and malformation with involucrum, cloaca, and sequestrum.[20–22,24] Osteomyelitis, an infection of both the cortex and marrow of bone, can be difficult to radiographically differentiate from infectious osteitis, an infection of the cortex only, because a lag separates clinical presentation and radiographic signs.[20,21,25] Some 30% to 60% of bone demineralizes before radiographic evidence of osteomyelitis is noted,[20,21,24,26,27] and 10 to 14 days of lag time separates the clinical disease and radiographic changes.[20,24,28] MRI, bone scintigraphy, and leukocyte-labeled scintigraphy (Indium-111, ^{99}mTc HMPAO) are valuable tools used in early diagnosis of osteomyelitis. MRI has demonstrated a sensitivity of 84% to 92% and a specificity of 84% in the diagnosis of osteomyelitis.[29–31] ^{99}Tc 3-phase bone scan demonstrates 90% to 100% sensitivity but less than 50% specificity.[29] In 1989, Seabold and colleagues[32] reported improvement in the specificity of ^{111}In-WBC imaging in the detection of osteomyelitis at fracture nonunion sites with the addition of ^{99m}Tc-MDP imaging by differentiating inflammation/infection in adjacent soft tissue from osteomyelitis at the fracture site. The gold standard of osteomyelitis diagnosis, however, remains the bone biopsy.[33]

It must be emphasized that no radiographic evaluation should replace clinical judgment or intraoperative evaluation, particularly in regard to the integrity of the syndesmosis and the presence or absence of bone infection. Radiographic findings should only be used as one component in the full depiction of a postsurgical complication, and should supplement preoperative clinical examination and intraoperative assessment.

FIBULAR MALUNION

Yablon and colleagues[5] demonstrated in 1977 the importance of the lateral malleolus in the anatomic reduction of bimalleolar fractures. After this in vitro and in vivo study, it was established that the displacement of the talus faithfully follows that of the lateral malleolus as a result of impingement of the lateral malleolus on the proximal fibular fragment. Only after adequate reduction of the lateral malleolus is achieved can the talus be anatomically repositioned. Malreduction of the distal fibula results in rotation and lateral shift of the talus with permanent instability and valgus tilt, in turn preventing the talus from being smoothly guided and supported between the malleoli and resulting in widening of the mortise, which may lead to posttraumatic arthritis.[34–36] In fact, in a majority of the symptomatic patients reported, it was found that there was incomplete reduction of the lateral malleolus and residual talar tilt.[37–39] More recently, according to Herscovici and colleagues[40] in 2008, three of the most common causes of persistent malreduction of pronation–external rotation (PER) injuries are inadequate restoration of fibular length, persistent external rotation of the fibula, and inadequate fixation of the fibula, as a result of use of a plate that is either too short or too malleable.

Residual displacement of the talus greatly reduces congruity and leads to degenerative changes as a result of reduction in contact area and therefore increase in localized contact pressure.[4,34,41–43] Specifically, decreased tibiotalar contact and increased localized lateral contact pressures were observed with fibular shortening, lateral shift of the fibula, and fibular external rotation, along with a divided deltoid ligament.[41,44]

Management

The restoration of the length and proper rotation of the fibula is an absolute priority. Even a minimal degree of shortening of the fibula indicates operative treatment. The successful use of internal fixation with fibular lengthening osteotomies has been reported.[7,11–13,45–48] Speed and Boyd[49] first reported that fibular osteotomy could correct shortening and external rotation. In 1976, Hughes[45] reported 28 cases of fibular shortening treated by a lengthening osteotomy. Results were good or better in 79%

of the reported 28 cases, with no correlation was found between the eventual outcome and initial method of treatment, the time to revision, or the age of the patient.

Offierski[11] reported a fair or good outcome in 91% of 11 patients who had fibular shortening treated with lengthening osteotomies, with the length of time to revision, the quality of reduction achieved, and the condition of the joint surface being the primary factors determining the success of the revision. In this study, it was reported that the age of the patient, the type of initial fibular fracture, and the initial treatment method did not affect the success of the revision. Weber and Simpson[7] reported, however, that the extent of arthritic change already present and the condition of the joint surface are much more important than the length of time since the initial injury or the amount of talar lateral displacement. In this study, no difference in outcomes was noted with the use of fibular lengthening osteotomies to correct overt and occult fibular malunions, as reported in 1989 by Yablon and Leach.[12]

When performing a lengthening osteotomy of the fibula, the distal fibula is exposed at the fracture site and scar tissue is excised. The previous incision is typically used, but could be extended anteriorly so that the anterior aspect of the tibiofibular joint and the interosseous membrane are exposed to allow for careful inspection. An oblique osteotomy of the lateral malleolus is performed at the level of the initial site of the fracture. A small distractor can be applied to the anterior surface of the fibula using two pairs of 2.5-mm threaded Kirschner wires, with the distal pair placed in 10° external rotation to provide the internal rotation of the distal fragment usually needed to correct the deformity, as described by Ward and colleagues[48] in 1990. Distraction is then used to restore the normal fibular length. Care must be taken with the distraction device to prevent twisting and torque on the distal screws, as suggested by Harper[50] in 1994. For mobile fibulae, a lamina spreader against either side of the fibula has been shown to provide adequate distraction.[51] The lateral malleolus may also be manually pulled distally and then internally rotated to reduce the subluxation of the joint. It is the primary author's preference, however, to use a small external fixator for temporary intraoperative distraction.

A corticocancellous graft can then be inserted in the resulting defect. For large defects, the corticocancellous graft from the iliac crest or calcaneus works well. The fibula can then be stabilized with a one-third tubular plate and a syndesmotic screw when necessary. A separate incision may also be made over the medial malleolus to remove the scar tissue between it and the medial wall of the talus if repositioning of the talus is difficult or if a widened medial clear space persists after fibular reduction. The talar reduction is also evaluated radiographically and assessed for corrected Shenton line of the ankle.

In the symptomatic patient who has advanced arthritic changes of the ankle joint, arthrodesis is indicated. To make this determination, whether or not patients are candidates for corrective fibular osteotomies, arthroscopy can be helpful. If arthroscopy demonstrates complete absence of articular cartilage in the tibial plafond or the talus, an arthrodesis is indicated. Marti and colleagues,[52] however, found few symptoms of arthritis after reconstruction and better tolerance of existing arthritis after correction of malalignment in a study averaging 7 years' follow-up.

Case Presentation

A 38-year-old male presented to the primary author's clinic with a complaint of right chronic ankle pain. The patient related having had sustained a "double" fracture of his right fibula 6 years prior which was subsequently close-reduced. The patient reported significant pain with active and passive ankle range of motion and on weightbearing, ambulation, and activity since the initial injury. Physical examination revealed pain on palpation at the area of the lateral malleolus and the lateral gutter of the ankle. Substantial decrease in the ankle range of motion was also noted.

Radiographic evaluation demonstrated significant fibular shortening, approximately 3 mm, as compared with the contralateral nonaffected extremity (**Fig. 1**A), with a difference of talocrural angles between extremities measured to be 8° (<2° deemed acceptable by Sarkisian and Cody).[10] Medial clear space was adequate (1–4 mm), as was the talar tilt (<1°), implying adequate syndesmotic reduction or absence of initial syndesmotic injury. Substantial degenerative changes were also clearly evident. Treatment options were discussed in detail with this patient, and the patient consented to undergo arthroscopic débridement of his ankle joint along with a fibular lengthening procedure. It was well depicted to the patient, however, and the patient thoroughly understood, that the primary goal of this procedure was to reduce his pain and that the prevention of continued arthrosis of his ankle joint was extremely unlikely.

Under general anesthesia with local infiltration, diagnostic and therapeutic ankle arthroscopy was first performed. A significant amount of hypertrophy and impingement synovitis was observed and débrided, as well as degenerative tissue and some chondromalacia at the lateral aspect of the ankle joint consistent with the previous fracture site.

Attention was then directed to the distal fibula, which was exposed through the previous incision. Substantial shortening and posterior malalignment of the distal portion of the fibula was observed intraoperatively. An oblique osteotomy of the lateral malleolus was performed at the level of the initial site of the fracture (see **Fig. 1**B) to allow for anterior and distal translocation of the distal fragment, so as to accommodate for shortening and posterior malalignment. Release of the syndesmosis was needed to allow for the fibular lengthening. A small uniplanar external fixator was placed on the lateral aspect of the fibula and was used for temporary intraoperative distraction (see **Fig. 1**C). A reduction forceps was placed on the lengthened fibula and two interfragmentary compression screws were placed across the fibula using standard arbeitsgemeinshaft osteosynthesefragen (AO) technique.

The bone clamp was removed, as was the external fixator, and length was noted to be held in position with an increase in length of approximately 5 mm. A fibular plate was placed on the lateral aspect of the fibula and fixation was accomplished with two screws superior and four screws distal to the fracture site. Because intraoperative evaluation of the syndesmosis revealed instability, a syndesmotic screw was placed through the plate to allow for syndesmotic stabilization. Intraoperative FluoroScan was used to verify adequate reduction of the fibula, and postoperative radiographs verifying adequate lengthening of the fibula with a talocrural angle comparable (<2°) to the contralateral extremity (see **Fig. 1**D, E). Ten weeks later, the patient returned to the OR for removal of the syndesmotic screw. The patient continues to have improved symptoms and reduced pain 1 year after the fibular lengthening osteotomy procedure.

FIBULAR NONUNION

The causes of nonunion have been well described: inadequate vascularity, instability, inadequate immobilization, poor bony contact, bone defects, and local infection. The initial injury can cause soft tissue stripping of the bone, which can damage the endosteal or periosteal blood supply, causing necrosis at the fracture site and eventual nonunion. Without adequate stabilization, excessive motion can cause widening at the fracture site and stimulate fibroblasts instead of osteoblasts, in turn resulting

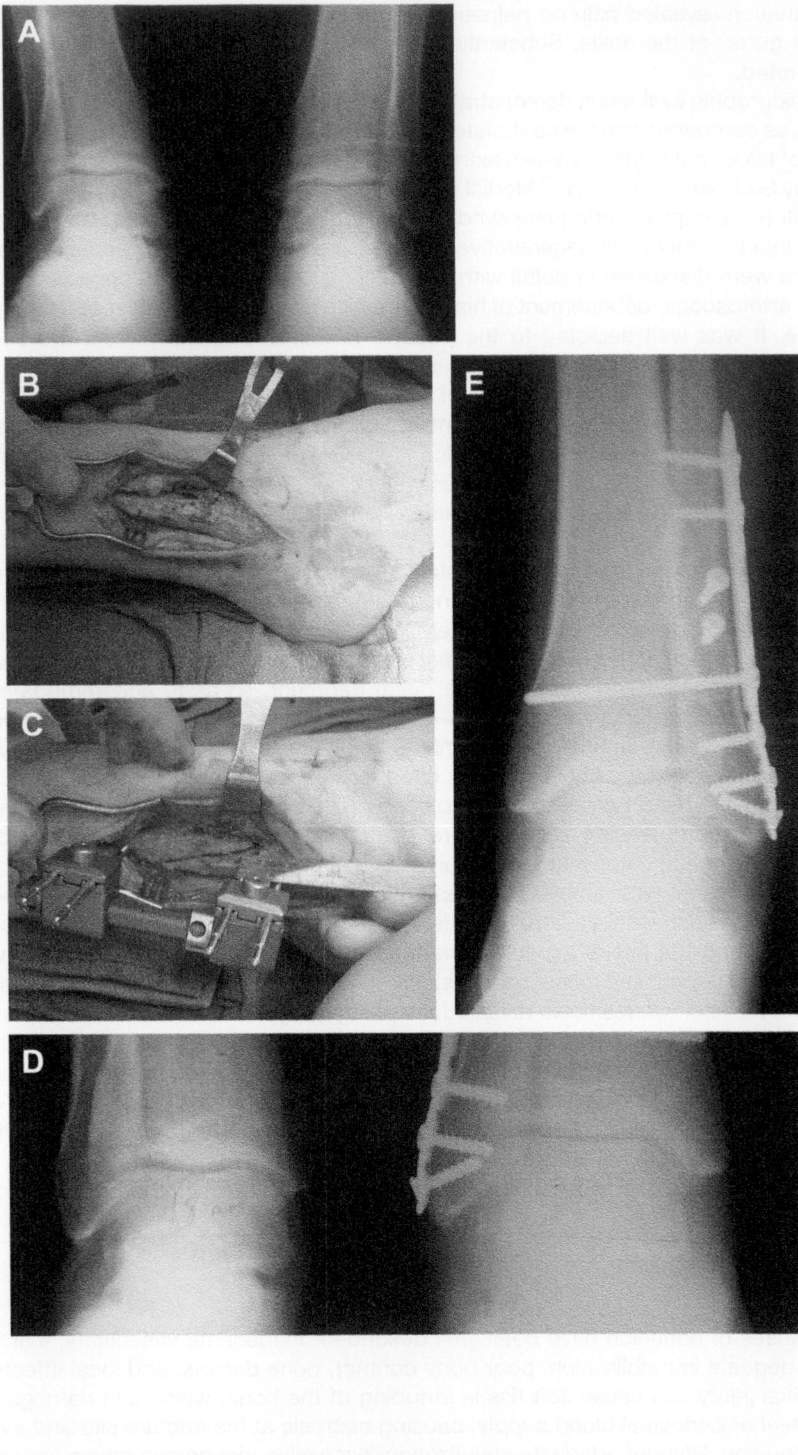
A
B
C
D
E

in fibrocartilage formation and subsequent nonunion.[53] The development of a nonunion generally is associated with pain, stiffness of surrounding joints, and disability.[54]

Management

The management of fibular nonunions is similar to the treatment of nonunions elsewhere, with the first step being the appropriate classification, namely the differentiation between hypertrophic (viable) and hypotrophic (nonviable) nonunions. Treatment of hypertrophic nonunions does not differ from that of delayed unions and consists of an extended immobilization period and internal fixation. Treatment of avascular nonunions, however, typically involves surgical intervention in the form of decortication or bone grafting.[15] Broadly, the important principles of treatment of hypertrophic and hypotrophic nonunions include the provision of stability, osteogenic potential, and control of infection.

MEDIAL MALLEOLAR MALUNION OR NONUNION

Open reduction of the lateral and medial malleoli is noted to be superior to closed reduction, but open reduction of only the medial malleolus has demonstrated worse results than closed reduction.[4] According to different authors, a pseudoarthrosis of the medial malleolus is considered a nonunion if not healed by 4 to 6 months.[55,56] Patients typically present with pain, instability, or persistent swelling that is related to the pseudarthrosis.

Management

Reconstruction of the medial malleolar fragment may be unpredictable, with one study reporting that only 50% of the medial malleolar nonunions treated with open reduction healed in osseous union.[57,58] For a small fractured medial malleolar fragment that does not contribute to the stability of the ankle joint, simple excision is appropriate. For larger fragments, principles described previously for lateral malleolar fractures apply, with recreation of the Shenton line of the ankle. Fixation can be achieved by using two partially threaded cancellous screws, cannulated screws, tension-banding techniques, or K-wire fixation, as long as two points of fixation are implemented. It is the authors' preference to use two partially-threaded cancellous screws, although tension-band wires have also been used successfully. The medial malleolus seldom needs a structural bone graft, because shortening is not a primary concern, as with the fibular malunions. As with nonunions elsewhere, however, supplementation with bone graft substitutes is advised.

Fig. 1. A 38-year-old male 6 years post reduction of a fibular fracture. (*A*) Radiographic evaluation demonstrating significant fibular shortening as compared with the contralateral extremity. (*B*) An oblique osteotomy of the lateral malleolus performed at the level of the initial site of the fracture to allow for anterior and distal translocation of the distal fragment, so as to accommodate for shortening and posterior malalignment. (*C*) Placement of a small uniplanar external fixator on the lateral aspect of the fibula to temporarily distract the fracture/osteotomy site intraoperatively. (*D*) Postoperative radiographs verifying adequate lengthening of the fibula with a talocrural angle comparable (<2°) to the contralateral extremity. (*E*) Intraoperative FluoroScan verifying adequate reduction of the fibula.

Case Presentation

A 35-year-old female presented to the primary author's clinic with the complaint of continued ankle pain 2 years after sustaining a supination external rotation (SER)–IV ankle fracture. The patient underwent ORIF of an ankle fracture 2 years prior, at which time the medial malleolar fracture was not addressed. CT evaluation confirmed the presence of a medial malleolar nonunion, with lack of trabeculation across the fracture site (**Fig. 2**A). After thorough discussion with the patient, it was determined that surgical reconstruction of the medial malleolar nonunion was the best treatment option.

The medial malleolus was exposed through the previous incision. A transverse arthrotomy of the medial malleolus was performed at the level of the initial site of the

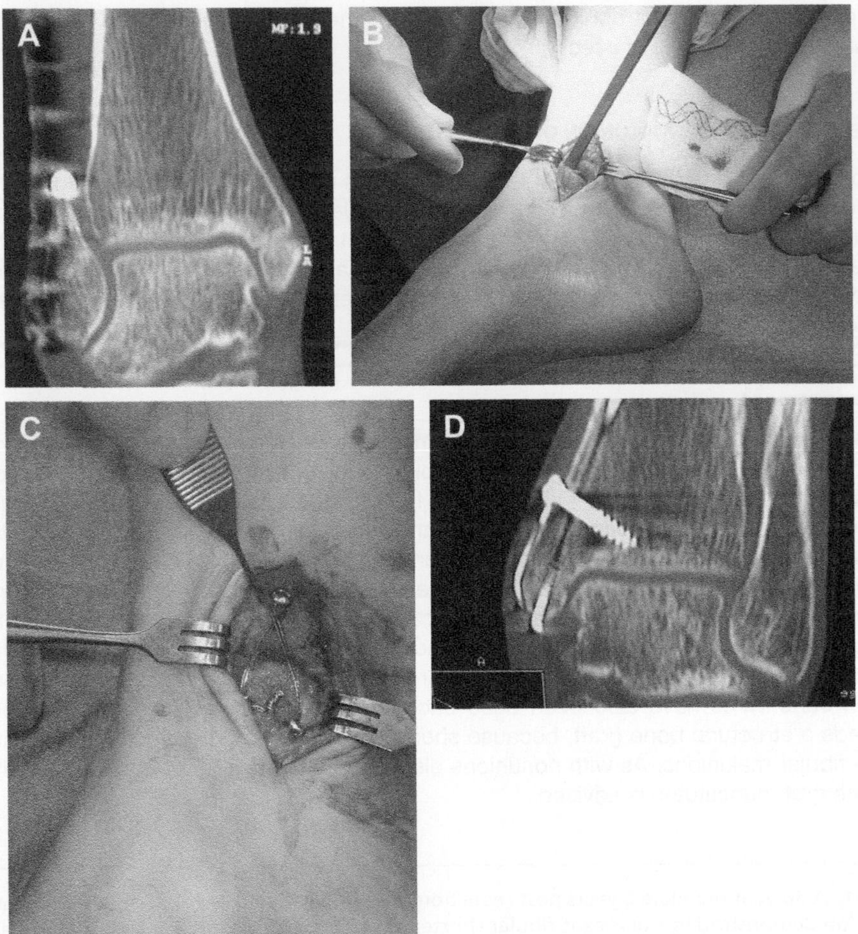

Fig. 2. A 35-year-old female 2 years post ORIF of an ankle fracture. (*A*) CT evaluation confirming the presence of a medial malleolar nonunion, with lack of trabeculation across the fracture site. (*B*) A transverse arthrotomy of the medial malleolus performed at the level of the initial site of the fracture using an osteotome. (*C*) Fixation of the fracture using a tension-banding technique. (*D*) CT obtained 12 weeks postreduction demonstrating a well-aligned reduction and appropriate healing across the medial malleolar fracture site.

fracture using an osteotome (see **Fig. 2**B). The fracture site was débrided substantially with use of a bone curette and rongeur, with excision of all remaining fibrotic tissue. Proper alignment of the fractured medial malleolar fragment on the tibia was obtained with use of a reduction forceps, with care taken to restore the medial articular surface. INFUSE (rhBMP-2) bone graft substitute was placed in the interface between the fracture site to supplement bone healing, and the fracture was fixated using a tension-banding technique (see **Fig. 2**C). Tension-band wires (70-mm and 90-mm) were placed across the medial malleolus and a 24-gauge wire and a 4.0-mm screw were placed superiorly to facilitate the locking portion. Figure-of-8 tension banding was accomplished, allowing for excellent compression across the medial malleolar nonunion site.

CT obtained at 12 weeks postreduction demonstrated a well-aligned reduction and appropriate healing across the medial malleolar fracture site (see **Fig. 2**D). The patient remains completely asymptomatic at her last follow-up, 4 years after the initial injury.

POSTERIOR MALLEOLAR NONUNION

Studies on trimalleolar fractures recommend reduction of a posterior malleolar fragment when it involves 25% of the articular surface or when it is markedly displaced with a 3-mm gap or 2-mm deformity.[58–60] These criteria are based on plain films and can be seen more clearly on CT scan. Posterior malleolar injuries rarely occur in isolation. Typically, they are associated with medial and lateral malleolar injuries. The posterior tibiofibular ligament, if intact, indirectly reduces the posterior malleolus with reduction of the fibula. In an evaluation of 306 cases of displaced ankle fractures treated surgically, Lindsjo[2] reported a significant increase in posttraumatic arthritis among cases with surface-bearing posterior fragments (34%), as compared with cases with small posterior fragments (17%) or cases without posterior fragments (4%). Mont and colleagues[8] also reported a worse result in patients who had a large posterior malleolar fracture (>20%). Harper and Hardin,[61] on the other hand, showed no clinical benefit from reducing the posterior malleolus after anatomic reduction of the medial and lateral malleoli.

Management

Malunited posterior malleolar fractures involving a relatively large portion of the articular surface also have marked talar malposition and severe arthritis.[16] These fractures are usually not amenable to reduction by way of osteotomies and normally require arthrodesis instead. If signs of degenerative joint changes are not yet evident, however, a posterior malleolar osteotomy could be performed through a posterior lateral incision after repositioning the fibula, as proposed by Mont and colleagues[8] in 1992. The posterior malleolus can then be fixated with an anterior-to-posterior screw or by direct fixation. Alternatively, the posterior malleolus can be reached posterior to the transfixed fibula and held with posterior-to-anterior screws. A posteromedial or posterolateral approach can be performed in revision cases in which the medial or lateral malleoli are intact. It is the authors' preference to fixate the posterior malleolar fragment with two anterior-to-posterior screws on initial ORIF or initial presentation. When addressing malunions or nonunions, it is the authors' preference to place the fixation directly from posterior to anterior to ensure proper reduction and compression.

Case Presentation

A 44-year-old female presented to the primary author's clinic with the complaint of continued ankle pain despite surgical treatment of a SER-IV type ankle fracture sustained 5 weeks prior. CT evaluation revealed a nonunion/malunion of the posterior malleolus with the fractured fragment encompassing 40% to 45% of the articular surface because of its significant elevation. This posterior malleolar fracture was not addressed during initial ORIF of the injury (**Fig. 3**A). In attempt to slow the progression of

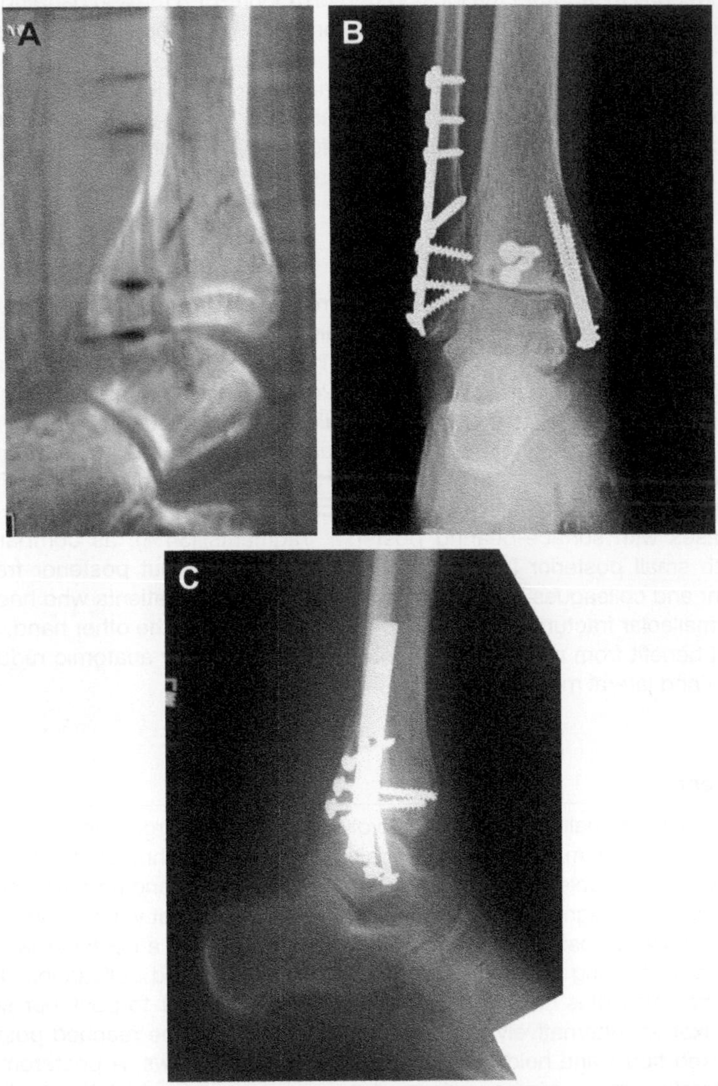

Fig. 3. A 44-year-old female 5 weeks post ORIF of an ankle fracture. (*A*) CT evaluation revealing a nonunion/malunion of the posterior malleolus with the fractured fragment encompassing 40% to 45% of the articular surface due to its significant elevation, which was not addressed during the initial procedure. (*B*, *C*) Postoperative radiographs demonstrating the use of two-point 4.0-mm cannulated screw fixation from posterior to anterior to prevent any rotation and to allow for compressive fixation of the now-reduced malunion.

the degenerative changes to the ankle joint and minimize the possibility of arthrosis long term, it was decided that surgical reconstruction of the posterior malunion be undertaken.

The posterior malleolus was exposed through a posterior-lateral incision, just lateral to the Achilles tendon. Care was taken not to damage the sural nerve. An extensive incision was necessary to fully expose the superior aspect of the fracture. A large osteotome was inserted at the superior fracture site and used to recreate the fracture. The fractured posterior malleolar fragment was mobilized, and proper alignment of the fragment on the tibia was obtained with use of a bone hook, with care taken to restore the tibial articular surface. Two-point 4.0-mm cannulated screw fixation from posterior to anterior was used to prevent any rotation and to allow for compressive fixation of the now-reduced malunion (see **Fig. 3**B, C). Postsurgically, the patient was immobilized nonweightbearing for 6 to 8 weeks. Aggressive physical therapy was prescribed because of significant postoperative stiffness, which was due to the immobilization from the initial fracture and the secondary immobilization. The patient healed uneventfully and was able to continue with her normal daily activities without significant limitations.

SYNDESMOTIC WIDENING

Adequate reduction of the tibiofibular syndesmosis in Weber B and C ankle fractures depends on proper reduction of the lateral malleolus. Adequate reduction of the syndesmosis and lateral malleolus correlates with good outcomes,[3] whereas failure to adequately reduce the syndesmosis is associated with posttraumatic arthritis and poorer outcomes.[18] Herscovici and colleagues[40] report that three of the most common causes of persistent malreduction of the syndesmosis are malreduction of one or both malleoli, osseous or soft tissue interposition, and malreduction of the fibula within the tibial incisura.

Management

Persistent or progressive widening of the syndesmosis, despite adequate reduction of the malleoli, can be treated with placement of a syndesmotic screw, if recognized early enough. It is the primary author's preference to use two 4.5-mm or 3.5-mm fully threaded cortical screws, through the fibular plate, if present. With PER-type fractures, stabilization across all four cortices is recommended. If persistent syndesmotic widening is present after removal of the syndesmotic screw or screws, reoperation is indicated. Anatomic reduction of the syndesmosis is necessary and scar formation should be induced by "roughing up" the anteromedial fibular soft tissues to change the biology of the region. The primary author does not routinely graft the syndesmosis, replace the syndesmotic ligament, or attempt a tibiofibular synostosis in primary repairs.

DEGENERATIVE CHANGES

The incidence of post-ORIF arthritis of the ankle is significantly greater in those fractures with postoperative displacement. Muller and colleagues[62] and Willenegger[63] found arthritis in 85.7% and 97%, respectively, of inadequately reduced fractures compared with 9.7% and 8%, respectively, of those accurately reduced. Overall incidences of postoperative arthritis range from 7.3% to 76%.[2,64] Lindsjö[2] reported a 14% incidence of posttraumatic arthritis of the ankle 2 to 6 years following open reduction, with middle-aged women being significantly more affected. Jarde and colleagues[65] reported degenerative changes in 37% of 32 ankles treated with internal fixation for fracture management and followed for at least 15 years, despite anatomic reconstruction. The authors of this series attributed the high incidence of arthritis to unrecognized injuries of the cartilaginous surfaces of the tibiotalar joint at the time of injury. The most common and most generally accepted criterion of arthritis is reduction of the joint space.[2]

Management

When severe degenerative changes are noted, the joint is often not worth reconstructing and an arthrodesis may be indicated. Arthroscopy can be used to determine the extent of articular disruption. If arthroscopy demonstrates complete absence of articular cartilage in the tibial plafond or the talus, an arthrodesis should be performed.

OSTEOMYELITIS/INFECTED NONUNION

The tibia is the most common site of bone infection, and osteomyelitis is not an uncommon complication of ORIF of ankle fractures. The presence of hardware further complicates the management because it often necessitates removal, leaving an unstable ankle complex. Infected nonunion has been defined as a failure of union and persistent infection at the fracture site for 6 to 8 months.[66] Although the open fracture is the most common cause of infected nonunion and the tibia is the most commonly involved bone, infected nonunion after implant surgery has nearly equal incidence, reportedly as a result of increased enthusiasm for operative fracture surgery.[67] Factors associated with nonunions include exposed bone devoid of vascularized periosteal coverage for more than 6 weeks, purulent discharge, a positive bacterial culture from the depth of the wound, and histologic evidence of necrotic bone containing empty lacunae.[68]

Management

The principles of treating osteomyelitis are well established and consist of aggressive débridement, infection control by intravenous antibiotics, stabilization, adequate soft tissue coverage, and management of skeletal defects if necessary.[69,70] Adequate débridement and eradication of necrotic tissue is the most important component of infection management and if not done thoroughly, bacteria sequestration would allow progression and recurrence of the disease.[71] Remaining hardware should be evaluated for loosening or lost maintenance of rigid fixation, and if noted, removal should be considered.[72] In the presence of stable internal fixation and evidence of response to local and systemic care, internal fixation may remain in place, with bone union given priority over the infection.[73] In addition to débridement and possible hardware removal, 4 to 6 weeks of intravenous antibiotics is recommended for patients who have osteomyelitis. Antibiotic-impregnated beads and spacers may also be used not only to provide high local concentrations of antimicrobial agents but also to assist in the management of skeletal dead space.[74,75]

Stabilization of the fracture or skeletal defect created after the resection of osteomyelitic bone is also of primary importance in the management of osteomyelitis, particularly if hardware must be removed and an unstable fracture remains. External fixation is the current method of choice for stabilization in this situation. Soft tissue coverage is also of vital importance, not only for coverage of exposed bone to prevent desiccation but also to improve the host defenses of the wound.[76–78] The vascularized muscle transfer improves host defenses at the wound site by providing oxygen and improving the host's own immune system at the infected site while obliterating the dead space.[76] Other ways of managing the skeletal defects created by the excision of infected or necrotic bone can be achieved with vascularized bone transfers,[79] autogenous bone grafting, and allografts, all of which can be supplemented with bone graft substitutes.

Case Presentation

A 46-year-old healthy male sustained a high fibular fracture (PER-type) as a result of a horse injury for which he was treated with ORIF. Four months after the surgical reduction of the fracture, the hardware reportedly broke and was therefore removed. At the time of hardware removal, an attempt to reconstruct the ensuing medial malleolar nonunion was performed. This procedure was complicated by an infection, for which the patient was treated with 6 weeks of intravenous vancomycin for the management of *Staphylococcus epidermidis*. Nine weeks after the hardware removal, he presented to the primary author's clinic with the complaint of continued drainage emanating from medial and lateral post-incisional wounds, and pain associated with his ankle despite the previous treatments. It was determined at this time that the remaining two medial screws should be removed because they might be contributing to residual infection.

Surgical débridement and curettage was performed by way of the previous medial and lateral incisions and the remaining two screws were removed from the medial malleolar nonunion site. Quantitative soft tissue cultures were obtained that confirmed the presence of continued infection with *S epidermidis*; a bone biopsy was obtained, which confirmed the presence of acute osteomyelitis. The wounds were thoroughly irrigated with pulsed lavage, the medial wound was packed with iodoform packing gauze, and the lateral dead space was packed with vancomycin- and gentamicin-impregnated methyl methacrylate antibiotic beads (**Fig. 4**A). Intraoperative evaluation confirmed the presence of soft and necrotic bone, loose fixation, and no or minimal healing at the medial and lateral malleolar fracture sites. The patient was placed on a 10-week course of intravenous antibiotics, followed by a 4-week course of oral antibiotics. A series of two operative débridements were performed over the next 2 weeks and a staged procedure was planned to reconstruct the resultant shortened fibula and the medial malleolar nonunion.

Sixteen weeks after initial débridement, a fibular-lengthening procedure was performed with the use of a calcaneal bicortical autogenous bone graft obtained from the patient's ipsilateral extremity. The previous lateral malleolar incision was used and upon intraoperative evaluation of the fibula, significant shortening of the fractured fragment was noted, as well as posterior displacement and valgus rotation of the fibula. Using a lamina spreader to distract the fracture site, the fibula was brought back to length (see **Fig. 4**B). Resection of nonviable bone was accomplished using a sagittal bone saw, leaving an approximately 0.25-in deficit. Pathologic evaluation of the specimen confirmed the absence of osteomyelitis. This deficit was replaced with an autogenous bicortical bone graft obtained from the calcaneus (see **Fig. 4**C), with supplementation with InFUSE (rhBMP-2) bone graft substitute. The defect created from retrieval of the calcaneus graft was filled with allogeneic bone chips. Temporary fixation of the fibula was afforded using a bone reduction forceps, and a 10-hole plate was placed on the lateral aspect of the fibula. The plate was fixated superiorly and distally with locking screws to help buttress the previous nonunion site. Two 3.5-mm fully threaded syndesmotic screws were placed across the distal portion of the plate.

The medial malleolar nonunion was reconstructed as described previously, with débridement of the fracture site, fixation using a tension-banding technique, and supplementation with INFUSE. The patient was placed empirically on intravenous

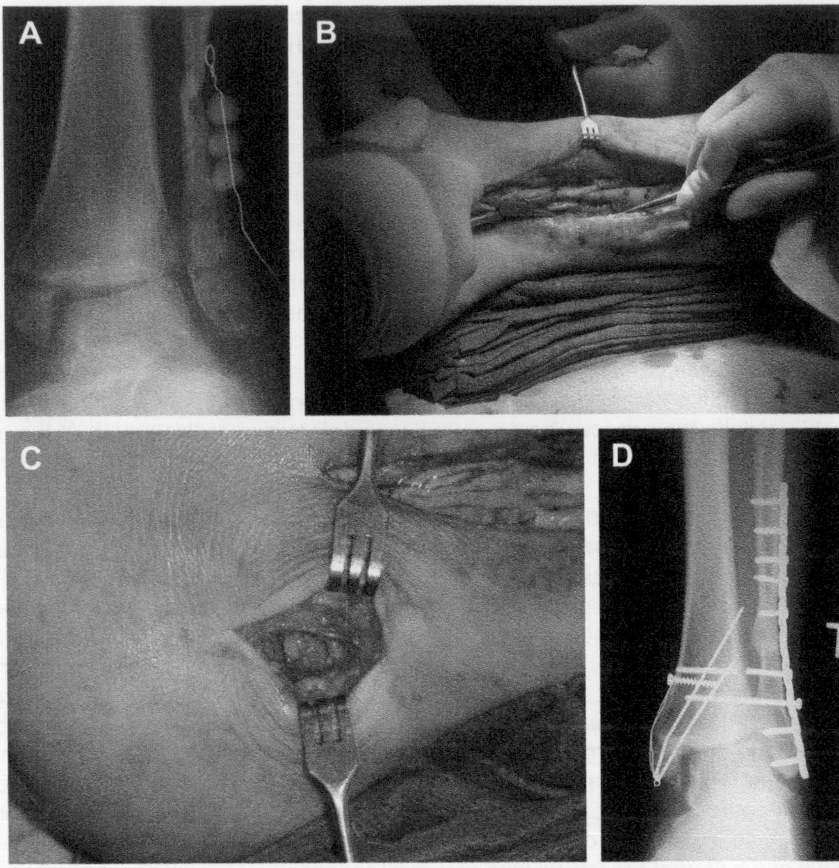

Fig. 4. A 46-year-old male 4 months post ORIF of a high fibular fracture. (*A*) Intraoperative FluoroScan demonstrating the removal of all hardware and the packing of the lateral dead space with vancomycin- and gentamicin-impregnated methyl methacrylate antibiotic beads, secondary to infected nonunions of the lateral and medial malleoli. (*B*) Sixteen weeks after initial débridement, a fibular lengthening procedure was performed. A lamina spreader was used to distract the fracture site and bring the fibula back to length. (*C*) The deficit created from the resection of all nonviable bone was replaced with an autogenous bicortical bone graft obtained from the calcaneus. (*D*) Radiographs obtained 6 months after reconstruction demonstrating osseous healing and extensive bone callus formation across the bone graft site.

vancomycin and imipenem. Radiographs obtained 6 months after reconstruction (see **Fig. 4**D) revealed osseous healing and extensive bone callous formation across the bone graft site. The patient went on to have the syndesmotic screws removed as a result of one breaking within the syndesmosis and further reconstruction of the medial malleolus as a result of a nonunion that was evidenced by hardware failure at the fracture site.

OSTEOMYELITIS WITH SEPTIC ANKLE ARTHRITIS

Treatment of distal tibial or fibular osteomyelitis with adjacent ankle sepsis poses a great challenge as a result of the decreased circulation of the overlying skin at this area, along with the resulting destruction of the ankle joint.[69] As with isolated osteomyelitis, the presence of hardware further complicates the management because it often necessitates removal, leaving an unstable ankle complex.

Management

Many authors propose ankle fusion in the presence of septic arthritis with concomitant chronic osteomyelitis.[69,80] In addition to eradication of the infection by thorough débridement and appropriate anti-infective management, emphasis is also placed on obtaining a biomechanically stable osteosynthesis.[80] Numerous techniques have been proposed for achieving ankle fusion in infected joints with concomitant osteomyelitis, including distraction osteogenesis using the Ilizarov technique,[81,82] free vascularized fibular autogenous bone grafting,[79] and delayed arthrodesis using autogenous bone graft and external fixation,[69,70] with or without free tissue transfers.[70,83–85] Fusion rates in the presence of ankle sepsis reportedly range from 71% to 87%,[80,81,86] as compared with aseptic ankle fusion rates of 88% to 100%.[87,88]

In 1989, Cierny and colleagues[86] proposed a single-staged procedure using a combination of bone grafting, external fixation, and osteocutaneous flaps, with a 21% failed fusion rate and a 22% primary amputation rate. On the basis of their results of more than 100 fusions of septic ankle joints, Cierny and Zorn[75] modified their approach in 1996 and recommended a staged reconstruction with temporary implantation of local antibiotics in cases with critical infections and large skeletal defects.

Different fixation techniques have been used successfully, including internal fixation, external fixation, and a combination of the two. Persistence of infection, as a result of implant loosening and reduction of bone stock, is a primary complication of internal fixation, whereas external fixation can result in pin track infections. External fixation is useful in maintaining stability in the presence of infection, particularly when internal hardware must be removed or a large defect remains after radical débridement of infected bone. In 1999, Richter and colleagues[80] proposed the use of both internal and external fixation, and reported a union rate of 86.6% in 45 patients. It was suggested in this study that titanium implants, which offer greater biocompatibility and less periosteal disturbance,[89–91] may be used in the presence of ongoing sepsis. Of their 45 patients, 20% did develop secretory fistulas with contact to the implants postoperatively, possibly because of the seeding of the infection with the screws. More recently, in 2003, Kollig and colleagues[92] reported a 93% fusion rate with the use of a "hybrid" external fixator consisting of Schanz screws in the tibial shaft and midfoot with fine titanium wires through the tarsal bones and the distal tibia. A biomechanical analysis of this system demonstrated comparable stability to a genuine ring fixator.[93] The authors prefer the use of external fixation only, with the circular fixator frame for a septic fusion.

Case Presentation

Four weeks after ORIF of a PER-IV ankle fracture (**Fig. 5**A), a 33-year-old male presented to the primary author's clinic with complaints of persistent fevers, chills, and night sweats for 2 to 3 days. On clinical evaluation, the ankle area was noted to be warm, swollen, and painful, with erythema extending proximally up the leg to the mid-calf level. The skin was intact with no purulence noted on initial presentation. The patient was admitted to the hospital with the diagnosis of septic arthritis and cellulitis. Emergent arthrotomy, débridement, and arthroscopic irrigation, using the ingress-egress technique, were performed with packing of open wounds. The patient was placed on intravenous antibiotics, and after three consecutive

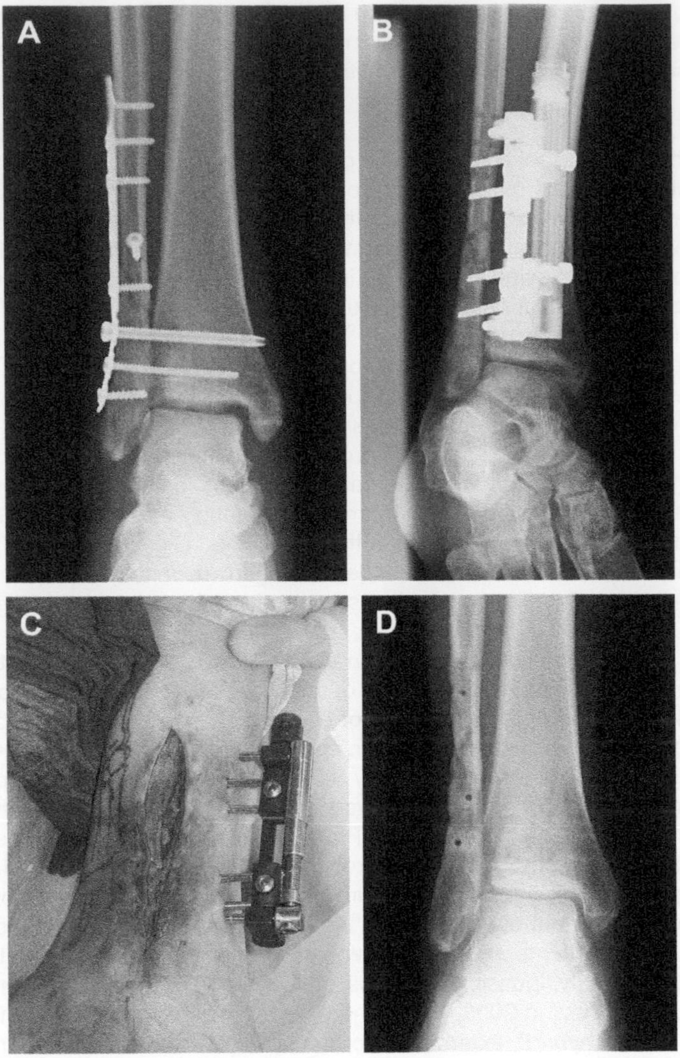

Fig. 5. A 33-year-old male 4 weeks post ORIF of an ankle fracture. (*A*) Radiographic evaluation obtained 4 weeks postoperatively when the patient presented with findings consistent with septic arthritis and lower extremity cellulitis. (*B, C*) Because the hardware was assumed to be acting as a nidus for continued infection, the fibular plate and screws were removed uneventfully, a soft tissue culture and a bone biopsy were obtained, and after thoroughly irrigating the wound, a uniplanar external fixator was applied to the anterior aspect of the fibula, proximal and distal to the fracture site, to stabilize the fracture. (*D*) Radiographic evaluation 10 weeks after fixator placement demonstrating trabeculations across the fracture site and osseous healing.

surgical irrigations and débridements and a 10-day hospital course, a significant improvement in cellulitis was noted and the wounds were closed primarily.

The patient was followed on an outpatient basis for several months, and after 3 months, no radiographic signs of healing were evident at the fibular fracture site. CT evaluation revealed evidence of fibular nonunion with signs of hardware loosening and possible infection, with the differential diagnosis being a fibular nonunion, and chronic osteomyelitis of the fibula. The remaining hardware was assumed to be acting as a nidus for continued infection. The risks were evaluated and it was decided to follow the infectious disease consultants' recommendations and remove the hardware. The fibular plate and screws were removed uneventfully, and a soft tissue culture and a bone biopsy were obtained. After after thoroughly irrigating the wound, a uniplanar external fixator was applied to the anterior aspect of the fibula, proximal and distal to the fracture site, to stabilize the fracture (see **Fig. 5**B, C). The external fixator remained in place for 12 weeks and radiographic evaluation 10 weeks after fixator placement revealed trabeculations across the fracture site and osseous healing (see **Fig. 5**D). The possibility of future ankle fusion was discussed in detail with the patient due to the liklihood of ensuing posttraumatic arthritis.

SUMMARY

The ankle is typically a resilient joint, but ankle fractures require accurate and immediate recognition, appropriate and complete diagnosis, and aggressive treatment. Radiographs must be evaluated thoroughly, with care taken to assess for fractures not only of the lateral malleolus but also of the medial and posterior malleoli. If pain ensues longer than expected after initial surgical correction, one must reassess for the presence of lateral, medial, and posterior malleolar malunions or nonunions, syndesmotic widening, and the possibility of degenerative changes to the ankle joint. Osteomyelitis and septic ankle arthritis are challenging complications, yet if recognized early and addressed appropriately and in a staged manner, excessive joint or bone destruction may be prevented. In all cases, the complications of surgical reduction must be thoroughly discussed with patients preoperatively. If the need for reconstruction arises postoperatively, the risks for continued degenerative joint changes and the possibility for ankle fusion in the future must be emphasized.

REFERENCES

1. de Souza LJ, Gustilo RB, Meyer TJ. Results of operative treatment of displaced external rotation-abduction fractures of the ankle. J Bone Joint Surg Am 1985; 67(7):1066–74.
2. Lindsjö U. Operative treatment of ankle fracture-dislocations. A follow-up study of 306/321 consecutive cases. Clin Orthop Relat Res 1985;199:28–38.
3. Pettrone FA, Gail M, Pee D, et al. Quantitative criteria for prediction of the results after displaced fracture of the ankle. J Bone Joint Surg Am 1983;65(5): 667–77.
4. Joy G, Patzakis MJ, Harvey JP Jr. Precise evaluation of the reduction of severe ankle fractures. J Bone Joint Surg Am 1974;56(5):979–93.
5. Yablon IG, Heller FG, Shouse L. The key role of the lateral malleolus in displaced fractures of the ankle. J Bone Joint Surg Am 1977;59(2):169–73.
6. Weber BG. Lengthening osteotomy of the fibula to correct a widened mortice of the ankle after fracture. Int Orthop 1981;4(4):289–93.
7. Weber BG, Simpson LA. Corrective lengthening osteotomy of the fibula. Clin Orthop Relat Res 1985;199:61–7.
8. Mont MA, Sedlin ED, Weiner LS, et al. Postoperative radiographs as predictors of clinical outcome in unstable ankle fractures. J Orthop Trauma 1992;6(3): 352–7.
9. Morris M, Chandler RW. Fractures of the ankle. Tech Orthop 1987;2(3):10–9.

10. Sarkisian JS, Cody GW. Closed treatment of ankle fractures: a new criterion for evaluation—a review of 250 cases. J Trauma 1976;16(4):323–6.
11. Offierski CM, Graham JD, Hall JH, et al. Late revision of fibular malunion in ankle fractures. Clin Orthop Relat Res 1982;171:145–9.
12. Yablon IG, Leach RE. Reconstruction of malunited fractures of the lateral malleolus. J Bone Joint Surg Am 1989;71(4):521–7.
13. Yablon IG. Occult malunion of ankle fractures—a cause of disability in the athlete. Foot Ankle 1987;7(5):300–4.
14. Sevitt S. Bone repair and fracture healing in man. New York: Churchill Livingstone; 1981.
15. Randolph TJ, Vogler H. Nonunions and delayed unions. J Foot Surg 1985;24:62–7.
16. Miller CD, Shelton WR, Barrett GR, et al. Deltoid and syndesmosis ligament injury of the ankle without fracture. Am J Sports Med 1995;23(6):746–50.
17. Close JR. Some applications of the functional anatomy of the ankle joint. J Bone Joint Surg Am 1956;38(4):761–81.
18. Leeds HC, Ehrlich MG. Instability of the distal tibiofibular syndesmosis after bimalleolar and trimalleolar ankle fractures. J Bone Joint Surg Am 1984;66(4):490–503.
19. Stiehl JB. Ankle fractures with diastasis. Instr Course Lect 1990;39:95–103.
20. Resnick D, Niwayama G. Diagnosis of bone and joint disorders. 2nd edition. Philadelphia: Saunders; 1988.
21. Edeiken J. Roentgen diagnosis of diseases of bone. Baltimore (MD): Williams & Wilkins; 1981.
22. Waldvogel FA, Medoff G, Swartz MN. Osteomyelitis: a review of clinical features, therapeutic considerations and unusual aspects N Engl J Med 1970;282(6):316–22.
23. Williams ML, Fleetor M. Radiographic evaluation of subacute osteomyelitis in children. Journal of Clinical Podiatric Medicine 1990;39(6):81–93.
24. Kehr LE, Zulli LP, McCarthy DJ. Radiographic factors in osteomyelitis. J Am Podiatry Assoc 1977;67(10):716–32.
25. Christman RA. The radiographic presentation of osteomyelitis in the foot. Clin Podiatr Med Surg 1990;7(3):433–48.
26. Bravo AA, Bruskoff BL, Perner R. A review of osteomyelitis with case presentation. J Am Podiatr Med Assoc 1985;75(2):83–9.
27. Bonakdapour A, Baines V. The radiology of osteomyelitis. Orthop Clin North Am 1983;14(1):21–37.
28. Schneider R, Freiberger RH, Ghelman B, et al. Radiologic evaluation of painful joint prostheses. Clin Orthop Relat Res 1982;170:156–68.
29. Frykberg RG. An evidence-based approach to diabetic foot infections. Am J Surg 2003;186(5A):44S–54S [discussion: 61S–4S].
30. Craig JG, Amin MB, Wu K, et al. Osteomyelitis of the diabetic foot: MR imaging-pathologic correlation. Radiology 1997;203(3):849–55.
31. Rosenberg ZS, Beltran J, Bencardino JT. From the RSNA refresher courses. Radiological Society of North America. MR imaging of the ankle and foot. Radiographics 2000;20(Spec No):S153–79.
32. Seabold JE, Nepola JV, Conrad GR, et al. Detection of osteomyelitis at fracture nonunion sites: comparison of two scintigraphic methods. AJR Am J Roentgenol 1989;152(5):1021–7.
33. Lipsky BA, Berendt AR, Deery HG, et al. Infectious Diseases Society of America. Diagnosis and treatment of diabetic foot infections. Clin Infect Dis 2004;39(7): 885–910.
34. Ramsey PL, Hamilton W. Changes in tibiotalar area of contact caused by lateral talar shift. J Bone Joint Surg Am 1976;58(3):356–7.

35. Brodie IA, Denham RA. The treatment of unstable ankle fractures. J Bone Joint Surg Br 1974;56(2):256–62.
36. Burwell HN, Charnley AD. The treatment of displaced fractures at the ankle by rigid internal fixation and early joint movement. J Bone Joint Surg Br 1965; 47(4):634–60.
37. Kleiger B. The treatment of oblique fractures of the fibula. J Bone Joint Surg Am 1961;43:969–79.
38. Magnusson R. On the late results in non-operated cases of malleolar fractures: clinical roentgenological-statistical study: fractures by external rotation. Acta Chir Scand 1944;(Suppl 84).
39. Solonen KA, Lauttamus L. Operative treatment of ankle fractures. Acta Orthop Scand 1968;39:223–37.
40. Herscovici D Jr, Anglen JO, Archdeacon M, et al. Avoiding complications in the treatment of pronation-external rotation ankle fractures, syndesmotic injuries, and talar neck fractures. J Bone Joint Surg Am 2008;90(4):898–908.
41. Lloyd J, Elsayed S, Hariharan K, et al. Revisiting the concept of talar shift in ankle fractures. Foot Ankle Int 2006;27(10):793–6.
42. Thordarson DB, Motamed S, Hedman T, et al. The effect of fibular malreduction on contact pressures in an ankle fracture malunion model. J Bone Joint Surg Am 1997;79(12):1809–15.
43. Moody ML, Koeneman J, Hettinger E, et al. The effects of fibular and talar displacement on joint contact areas about the ankle. Orthop Rev 1992;21(6):741–4.
44. Curtis MJ, Michelson JD, Urquhart MW, et al. Tibiotalar contact and fibular malunion in ankle fractures. A cadaver study. Acta Orthop Scand 1992;63(3):326–9.
45. Hughes JL. Corrective osteotomies of the fibula after defectively healed ankle fractures. J Bone Joint Surg Am 1976;58:728–35.
46. Marti R, Gitz H. Late reconstruction of malunited fractures of the ankle. Proceedings of SICOT 6th Congress, London: 1984:17.
47. Weller S, Knapp U, Eck T. Results of corrective operations of the ankle joint. In: Weller S, Hierholzer G, Hermichen HG, editors. Late results after osteosynthesis—collective results. Tubingen: AO International; 1984. p. 169–73.
48. Ward AJ, Ackroyd CE, Baker AS. Late lengthening of the fibula for malaligned ankle fractures. J Bone Joint Surg Br 1990;72(4):714–7.
49. Speed JS, Boyd HB. Operative reconstruction of malunited fractures about the ankle joint. J Bone Joint Surg 1936;18:270–86.
50. Harper MC. Malunited ankle fracture alignment. In: Johnson RA, editor. The foot and ankle. New York: Raven Press; 1994. p. 451–65.
51. Mast J, Jacob R, Ganz R. Planning and reduction techniques in fracture surgery. New York: Springer-Verlag; 1989.
52. Marti RK, Raaymakers EL, Nolte PA. Malunited ankle fractures. The late results of reconstruction. J Bone Joint Surg Br 1990;72(4):709–13.
53. Browner B, Jupiter J, Levine A, et al. Skeletal trauma basic science management and reconstruction. 3rd edition. Philadelphia: WB Saunders; 2003. p. 507–10.
54. Borrelli J Jr, Prickett WD, Ricci WM. Treatment of nonunions and osseous defects with bone graft and calcium sulfate. Clin Orthop Relat Res 2003;411:245–54.
55. Stiehl JB. Late reconstruction of ankle fractures and dislocations. In: Gould JS, editor. Operative foot surgery. Philadelphia: WB Saunders; 1994. p. 356–76.
56. Thomas RH, Daniels TR. Ankle arthritis. J Bone Joint Surg Am 2003;85(5): 923–36.
57. Sneppen O. Treatment of pseudarthrosis involving the malleolus. A postoperative follow-up of 34 cases. Acta Orthop Scand 1971;42(2):201–16.

58. Rockwood CA, et al. Fractures in adults, vol. 2. Philadelphia: Lippincott-Raven; 1996.
59. McDaniel WJ, Wilson FC. Trimalleolar fractures of the ankle. An end result study. Clin Orthop Relat Res 1977;122:37–45.
60. McLaughlin HL, Ryder CT Jr. Open reduction and internal fixation for fractures of the tibia and ankle. Surg Clin North Am 1949;29(4):1523–34.
61. Harper MC, Hardin G. Posterior malleolar fractures of the ankle associated with external rotation-abduction injuries. Results with and without internal fixation. J Bone Joint Surg Am 1988;70(9):1348–56.
62. Muller ME, Allgower M, Schneider R. Manual of internal fixation: techniques recommended by the AO Group. 2nd edition. Berlin: Springer-Verlag; 1979.
63. Willenegger H. Treatment of luxation fractures of the tibiotarsal joint according to biomechanical viewpoints. Helv Chir Acta 1961;28:225–39.
64. Day GA, Swanson CE, Hulcombe BG. Operative treatment of ankle fractures: a minimum ten-year follow-up. Foot Ankle Int 2001;22(2):102–6.
65. Jarde O, Vives P, Havet E, et al. Malleolar fractures. Predictive factors for secondary osteoarthritis. Retrospective study of 32 cases. Acta Orthop Belg 2000;66(4): 382–8.
66. Meyer S, Weiland AJ, Willenegger H. The treatment of infected non-union of fractures of long bones. Study of sixty-four cases with a five to twenty-one-year follow-up. J Bone Joint Surg Am 1975;57(6):836–42.
67. Toh CL, Jupiter JB. The infected nonunion of the tibia. Clin Orthop Relat Res 1995;315:176–91.
68. Jain AK, Sinha S. Infected nonunion of the long bones. Clin Orthop Relat Res 2005;431:57–65.
69. Thordarson DB, Ahlmann E, Shepherd LE, et al. Sepsis and osteomyelitis about the ankle joint. Foot Ankle Clin 2000;5(4):913–28.
70. Thordarson DB, Patzakis MJ, Holtom P, et al. Salvage of the septic ankle with concomitant tibial osteomyelitis. Foot Ankle Int 1997;18(3):151–6.
71. Waldvogel FA, Papageorgiou PS. Osteomyelitis: the past decade. N Engl J Med 1980;303(7):360–70.
72. McNeur JC. The management of open skeletal trauma with particular reference to internal fixation. J Bone Joint Surg Br 1970;52(1):54–60.
73. Lifeso RM, Al-Saati F. The treatment of infected and uninfected non-union. J Bone Joint Surg Br 1984;66(4):573–9.
74. Cierny G, Zorn KE. Arthrodesis of the tibiotalar joint for sepsis. Foot Ankle Clin 1996;1:177–97.
75. Klemm K. The use of antibiotic-containing bead chains in the treatment of chronic bone infections. Clin Microbiol Infect 2001;7(1):28–31.
76. Chang N, Mathes SJ. Comparison of the effect of bacterial inoculation in musculocutaneous and random-pattern flaps. Plast Reconstr Surg 1982;70(1): 1–10.
77. Boeckx W, van den Hof B, van Holder C, et al. Changes in donor site selection in lower limb free flap reconstructions. Microsurgery 1996;17(7):380–5.
78. Moore JR, Weiland AJ. Free vascularized bone and muscle flaps for osteomyelitis. Orthopedics 1986;9(6):819–24.
79. Bishop AT, Wood MB, Sheetz KK. Arthrodesis of the ankle with a free vascularized autogenous bone graft. Reconstruction of segmental loss of bone secondary to osteomyelitis, tumor, or trauma. J Bone Joint Surg Am 1995;77(12):1867–75.
80. Richter D, Hahn MP, Laun RA, et al. Arthrodesis of the infected ankle and subtalar joint: technique, indications, and results of 45 consecutive cases. J Trauma 1999; 47(6):1072–8.

81. Hawkins BJ, Langerman RJ, Anger DM, et al. The Ilizarov technique in ankle fusion. Clin Orthop Relat Res 1994;303:217–25.
82. Johnson EE, Weltmer J, Lian GJ, et al. Ilizarov ankle arthrodesis. Clin Orthop Relat Res 1992;280:160–9.
83. Patzakis MJ, Abdollahi K, Sherman R, et al. Treatment of chronic osteomyelitis with muscle flaps. Orthop Clin North Am 1993;24(3):505–9.
84. Patzakis MJ, Mazur K, Wilkins J, et al. Septopal beads and autogenous bone grafting for bone defects in patients with chronic osteomyelitis. Clin Orthop Relat Res 1993;295:112–8.
85. Patzakis MJ, Scilaris TA, Chon J, et al. Results of bone grafting for infected tibial nonunion. Clin Orthop Relat Res 1995;315:192–8.
86. Cierny G III, Cook WG, Mader JT. Ankle arthrodesis in the presence of ongoing sepsis. Indications, methods, and results. Orthop Clin North Am 1989;20(4): 709–21.
87. Scranton PE Jr. Use of internal compression in arthrodesis of the ankle. J Bone Joint Surg Am 1985;67(4):550–5.
88. Mann RA, Rongstad KM. Arthrodesis of the ankle: a critical analysis. Foot Ankle Int 1998;19(1):3–9.
89. Barth E, Myrvik QM, Wagner W, et al. In vitro and in vivo comparative colonization of Staphylococcus aureus and Staphylococcus epidermidis on orthopaedic implant materials. Biomaterials 1989;10(5):325–8.
90. Matter P, Burch HB. Clinical experience with titanium implants, especially with the limited contact dynamic compression plate system. Arch Orthop Trauma Surg 1990;109(6):311–3.
91. Pfeiffer KM, Brennwald J, Büchler U, et al. Implants of pure titanium for internal fixation of the peripheral skeleton. Injury 1994;25(2):87–9.
92. Kollig E, Esenwein SA, Muhr G, et al. Fusion of the septic ankle: experience with 15 cases using hybrid external fixation. J Trauma 2003;55(4):685–91.
93. Lundy DW, Albert MJ, Hutton WC. Biomechanical comparison of hybrid external fixators. J Orthop Trauma 1998;12(7):496–503.

Revisional Charcot Foot and Ankle Surgery

John J. Stapleton, DPM, AACFAS[a], Ronald Belczyk, DPM, AACFAS[b], Thomas Zgonis, DPM, FACFAS[b,*]

KEYWORDS

- Charcot foot • Diabetic neuropathy • Diabetic limb salvage
- Revisional foot and ankle surgery • Ilizarov external fixation

RATIONALE FOR SURGICAL INTERVENTION

Certainly not all patients who have Charcot deformities require surgical reconstruction. Many can be effectively managed with proper shoe modifications, orthoses, or bracing. Surgical treatment is indicated for ambulatory patients with recurrent ulceration, unstable scar formation, deep infection, unstable and unbraceable deformities, or chronic pain, however. The goal of operating on a Charcot deformity is to provide the patient with a functional limb that is stable, mechanically sound, and resistant to further skin breakdown while resuming an ambulatory status.[1–4] Reconstructive surgery for Charcot deformities can be quite challenging for the surgeon because of severe irreducible and unstable fractures and dislocations, poor bone quality, infection, and soft tissue compromise.[5]

Revisional cases are even more difficult secondary to inherent conditions, such as scar contractures, nonhealing incisions, further disuse osteopenia, vascular injury, bone loss, nonunions, deep infection, and failed fixation methods. The overall complication rate after surgical intervention for the Charcot foot and ankle varies widely in the literature; however, it is generally thought that patients who have diabetic neuropathy have higher rates of complications.[6] Stuart and Morrey[6] reported a 78% complications rate of neuropathic arthropathy in the failure of ankle arthrodesis, which included nonunions, deep infections, and below-the-knee amputations. As far as revisional surgery for Charcot deformities is concerned, there is little in the literature regarding the management of surgical failures. Unfortunately, surgical complications in the presence of Charcot neuroarthropathy (CN) are often managed with a major limb amputation. At times, a major limb amputation may be warranted or preferred, but alternative surgical procedures and techniques may be useful in the surgeon's armamentarium in managing these difficult revisional cases. The surgical management of Charcot

[a] Foot and Ankle Surgery, VSAS Orthopaedics, Allentown, PA, USA
[b] Department of Orthopaedic Surgery, Division of Podiatric Medicine and Surgery, The University of Texas Health Science Center, San Antonio, TX, USA
* Corresponding author. 7703 Floyd Curl Drive/MCS 7776, San Antonio, TX 78229, USA.
E-mail address: zgonis@uthscsa.edu (T. Zgonis).

Clin Podiatr Med Surg 26 (2009) 127–139
doi:10.1016/j.cpm.2008.09.004
podiatric.theclinics.com
0891-8422/08/$ – see front matter

deformities is associated with a steep learning curve, and complications are commonly encountered by inexperienced surgeons. This article reviews some of the challenges associated with revisional surgery, discusses potential reasons for surgical failure in patients who have diabetes mellitus and peripheral neuropathy, and, finally, provides some considerations for revisional Charcot reconstruction and limb salvage procedures.[7]

Principles Associated with Revisional Charcot Foot and Ankle Surgery

Establishing a treatment plan for revisional Charcot foot and ankle surgery begins with defining the current issues that need to be addressed, with a time frame for each, while addressing the factors that might have led to surgical failure during the initial operation. Typically, the goals of revisional surgery are different from or perhaps more complicated than those of the initial procedure. There are many potential reasons for treatment failures in the management of Charcot deformities. Those discussed in further detail include the following: missing the correct diagnosis initially, mechanical failure of hardware, recurrent deformity with or without ulceration, appropriately addressing the role of Achilles tendon lengthening, and soft tissue infection with or without concomitant osteomyelitis. Neuropathic osteoarthropathy has been reported by some researchers to contribute to an increased number of complications and failure rates.[1–6] Because revisional surgery may involve multiple complicating issues, a stepwise rationale approach, along with a strong understanding of the timing of surgery, is essential for the patient's successful outcome.

As with any revisional case, a thorough history and physical examination; review of chart records, previous radiographs and imaging studies, operative reports, and laboratory studies; and discussion with the prior treating physicians can give additional insight into the events that led up to a poor surgical outcome. Careful preoperative evaluation and patient selection are fundamental to reduce the risks associated with future surgery. Neglecting such issues as patient compliance and psychosocial issues leads to further complications regardless of the surgical plan. Awareness of patient-related variables that may increase the risks for complications should allow for better preoperative planning and overall management of the patient.

Surgical considerations for the management of failed Charcot intervention mostly depend on the underlying pathologic findings. Often, there are a multitude of factors that lead to poor outcomes, and the treatment approach for revisional surgery is not completely straightforward. The recommendations given here address five major categories that can lead to surgical complications and, at times, limb loss if not appropriately addressed.

Inaccurate initial diagnosis and the "pre-Charcot patient"

If the initial diagnosis of peripheral neuropathy and the loss of protective sensation were not made and the patient was not aggressively immobilized after foot or ankle surgery, a cascade of events can eventually follow, leading to neuropathic fractures, dislocations, and a worsening deformity. The most important factor in potentially altering the outcome of patients who have CN is to have a high clinical suspicion in patients who are "at risk." The surgeon needs to consider, treat, and educate the "pre-Charcot" patient, who can be defined as the patient with a loss of protective sensation detected by a 5.07 monofilament. Similarly, the patient who has diabetic neuropathy and has undergone surgery needs to be treated as a pre-Charcot patient and immobilized 59% longer than the sensate patient and with protective and monitored weight bearing once permitted.

A common example is the diabetic patient who has peripheral neuropathy and has sustained a low-energy ankle fracture that has been treated with open reduction internal fixation. Typically, these patients are allowed weight bearing for 6 to 8 weeks after surgery. Patients who have peripheral neuropathy and loss of protective sensation may need to be immobilized 9 to 12 weeks, however, along with evidence of radiographic healing of the fracture(s), before a protected partial to full weight-bearing status is initiated. This case scenario is seen frequently in the authors' practices, and the end result of the acute Charcot joint(s) is often misdiagnosed and untreated, which further complicates the proposed revisional limb salvage surgery. Common misdiagnoses include an infectious process or deep vein thrombosis as opposed to an acute Charcot joint; therefore, the cascade of events continues to occur because the patients are ambulating unprotected during the initial Charcot process.

Neuropathic fractures of the foot in patients who have diabetes are often triggered by an unrealized physical insult.[8,9] Up to 50% of patients who present with CN do not recall a history of trauma. Associated diabetic comorbidities, such as obesity, retinopathy, nephropathy, osteoporosis, and a loss of balance also contribute to additional risks for traumatic events in the postoperative period. This results in inadequate treatment, allowing for continued ambulation on a deteriorating foot and the destruction of foot architecture.[10] Although the exact prevalence of Charcot deformity is unknown, it is estimated that 1 in 680 patients who have diabetes develops Charcot deformity and that it affects 29% of diabetics who have peripheral neuropathy.[11] Subjective and objective pain scales simply cannot be applied to the neuropathic patient after surgery. As treating physicians, we need to identify pre-Charcot patients before their initial reconstruction and alter their treatment regimens accordingly to prevent any further future surgical complications.

Mechanical failure of hardware

A commonly encountered complication in the management of revisional Charcot surgery relates to the mechanical failure of various fixation methods. The most common cause of hardware failure or breakage is delayed osseous healing. Other reasons for hardware failure are poor bone quality, early weight bearing, noncompliance, inadequate fixation methods, poor surgical technique, and infection.

Internal fixation can only withstand so much mechanical stress and fatigue before the threshold is met and breakage occurs. There are various characteristics beyond the scope of this article that are involved in the design of internal fixation and lead to its overall mechanical strength. The surgeon operating on patients who have complex CN needs to have a great understanding of their diminished cortical stiffness and poor bone quality, and thus an ability to choose the most appropriate form of fixation to achieve a successful outcome depending on the anatomic location, procedure selected, and presence of soft tissue compromise.

Poor bone quality may be secondary to endocrine and renal abnormalities. Renal abnormalities in patients who have diabetes affect bone remodeling. Renal osteodystrophy in this patient population is partially attributable to a lack of dietary calcium intake, a lack of production of vitamin D, increased absorption of calcium from bone, and decreased excretion of phosphate from the kidneys. Hence, poor biology may predispose a patient to a poor outcome if the method of fixation fails before osseous consolidation. Medical management of osteoporosis supplemented by nutritional support can only be beneficial in the overall patient's successful outcome. In addition, revisional Charcot surgery is usually performed 6 months to years after the initial surgery and after the patient has been immobilized or non–weight bearing for a significant period of time, which may lead to further generalized disuse osteopenia. Conversely,

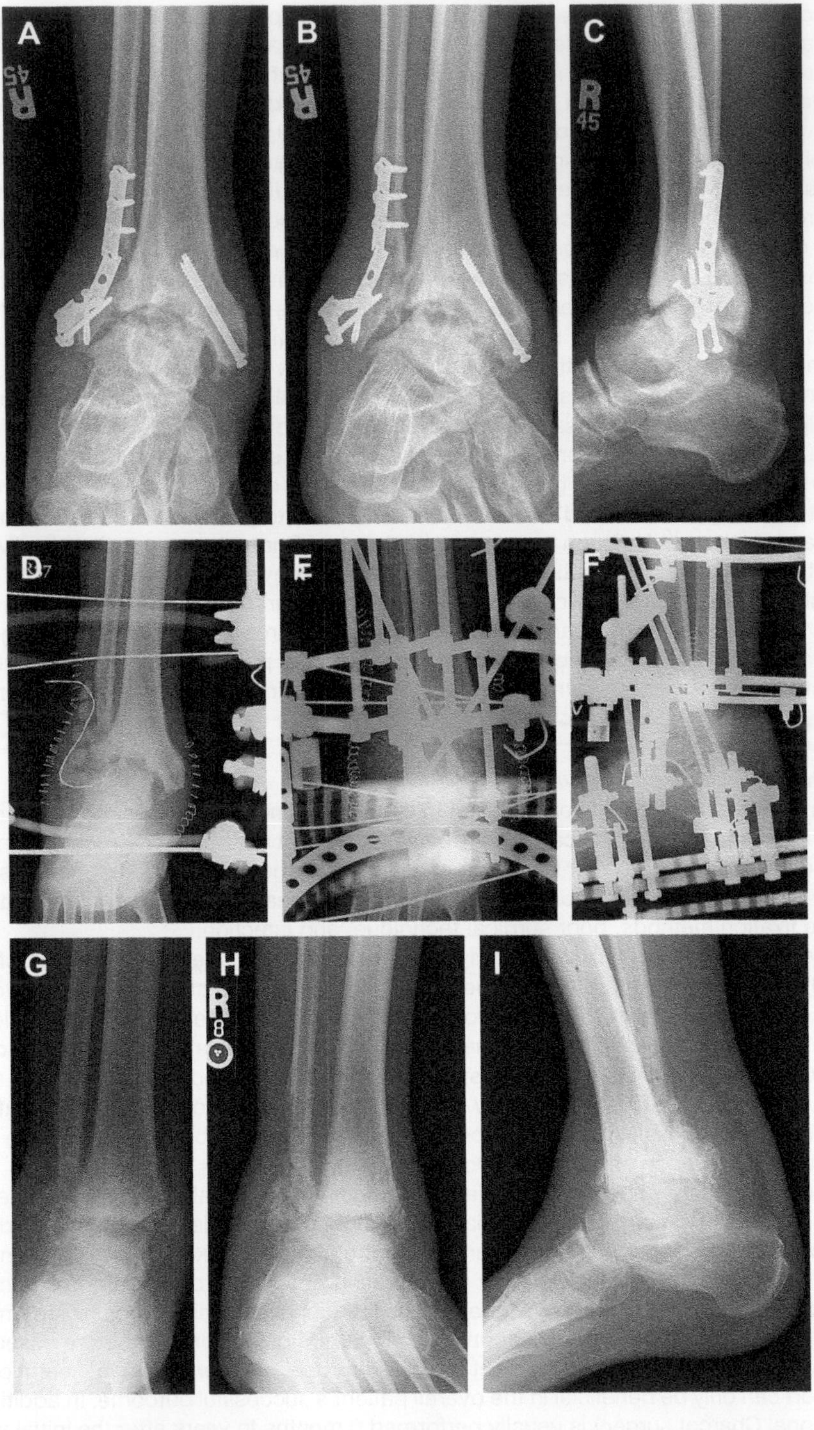
A
B
C
D
E
F
G
H
I

urgent or emergent revisional Charcot surgery is initiated immediately in the presence of a severe limb or life-threatening postoperative infection (**Fig. 1**).

The complications and inherent difficulty of using internal fixation in CN have been well documented. Shibata and colleagues[12] preferred the intramedullary nail with staples or Kirschner wires to control rotation because rigid internal fixation with plates or screws could not be used in patients who have leprotic neuroarthropathy as a result of osteoporotic bone and the danger that prominent screw heads may have caused necrosis of the overlying skin. Currently, the reconstructive surgeon has more options for preventing hardware failure in the surgical management of patients who have CN as new advances in internal and external fixation continue to occur. Technologic advances, such as locking plating systems, anatomically designed intramedullary rods, and circular external fixation systems, are an essential part of the surgeon's armamentarium in the management of revisional Charcot surgery.

Surgical techniques to prevent hardware failure include the incorporation of nonessential joints to obtain better fixation or extended joint arthrodesis procedures to obtain successful osseous union. These surgical techniques are commonly used and cannot be overlooked to achieve salvage of previous hardware failure. Some examples include but are not limited to the following: (1) placement of fibula-tibia screws in the management of diabetic neuropathic ankle fractures when possible, (2) columnar beaming after removal of an external fixator if further instability is suspected after attempted medial or lateral column arthrodesis procedures, (3) pantalar arthrodesis to control severe hindfoot and ankle deformities, and (4) extended medial or lateral column arthrodesis for management of failed isolated arthrodesis procedures. Furthermore, circular external fixation offers increased osseous stability while providing compression to achieve successful revisional joint arthrodesis. It is also ideal in cases of severe bone loss, soft tissue infection, osteomyelitis, and bony nonunion.

Immobilization immediately after the initial reconstructive surgery is critical in preventing hardware failure, but strict adherence to a non–weight-bearing status is often unreasonable in the patient who is obese, has vision complications, or has a lack of sensation. Postoperative recommendations vary in the literature from early immobilization to prolonged non–weight bearing. This also varies based on the type of fixation used. Wang and colleagues[13] proposed that the use of external fixation with bone stimulation may be an effective alternative method of treating the Charcot foot. Most patients were weight bearing in 10 to 14 days.

In summary, methods of fixation and close postoperative monitoring may prevent or identify future complications as soon as they occur. Based on the authors' experience, it is helpful to double the amount of fixation when internal fixation is used; use external fixation with poor bone stock, infection, or soft tissue compromise; increase the length

Fig. 1. (*A–C*) Radiographs show a failed bimalleolar ankle fracture repair with internal fixation 7 weeks after the original operation. This patient who had diabetic neuropathy and an ankle fracture presented with an infected ankle joint and signs of a pre-Charcot disease. He was immediately admitted to the hospital for a bone and soft tissue biopsy and removal of hardware. (*D*) Positive cultures necessitated the use of antibiotic beads and a hybrid external fixation for joint stability and close monitoring of the partially open wounds. (*E–F*) Eight weeks later, the patient was eventually brought back to the operating room for removal of the hybrid frame and antibiotic beads, further bone biopsy, and final ankle fusion with the use of Ilizarov external fixation. The Ilizarov external fixator was kept for 10 weeks. (*G–I*) All incisions eventually healed, and the patient maintained a clinically stable ankle for an accommodative ankle-foot-orthosis device.

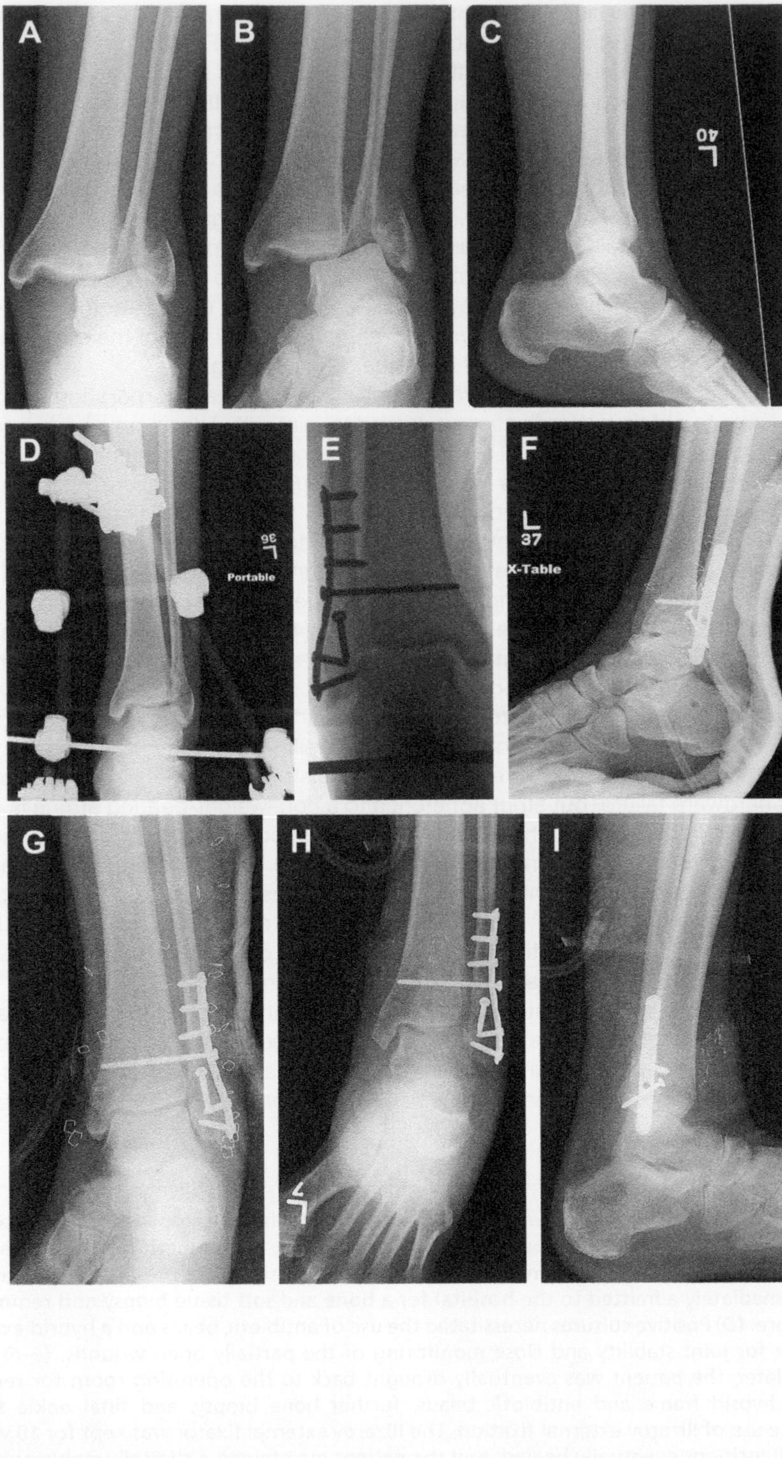
A
B
C
D
Portable
E
F
L
37
X-Table
G
H
I

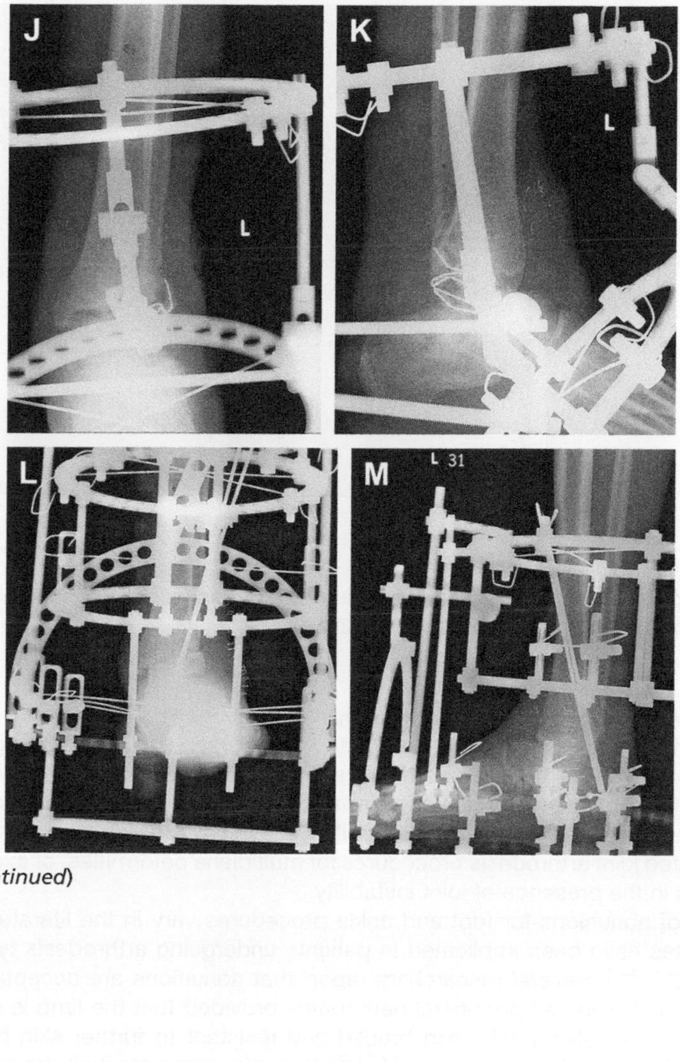

Fig. 2. (*continued*)

Fig. 2. Severely open dislocated ankle (*A–C*) was immediately spanned and reduced with a delta frame at initial presentation (*D*). (*E–I*) This patient who had diabetic neuropathy was brought back to the operating room within 5 days after the initial injury for an open reduction and internal fixation, followed by the use of a gracilis free flap after the ankle stabilization. Three months after the initial operation, the patient was referred with an infected ankle joint and signs of a pre-Charcot disease. He was immediately admitted to the hospital for bone and soft tissue biopsies and removal of hardware. (*J–K*) Positive cultures necessitated the use of antibiotic beads and a hybrid external fixation for joint stability and close monitoring of the partially open wounds. (*L–M*) Nine weeks later, the patient was eventually brought back to the operating room for removal of the hybrid frame and antibiotic beads, further bone biopsy, and final ankle fusion with the use of Ilizarov external fixation and an autogenous iliac crest bone grafting for realignment and solid bony union. (*N–P*) Ilizarov external fixator was kept for 12 weeks. All incisions eventually healed, and the patient maintained a clinically stable ankle in a slight valgus position for an accommodative ankle-foot-orthosis device.

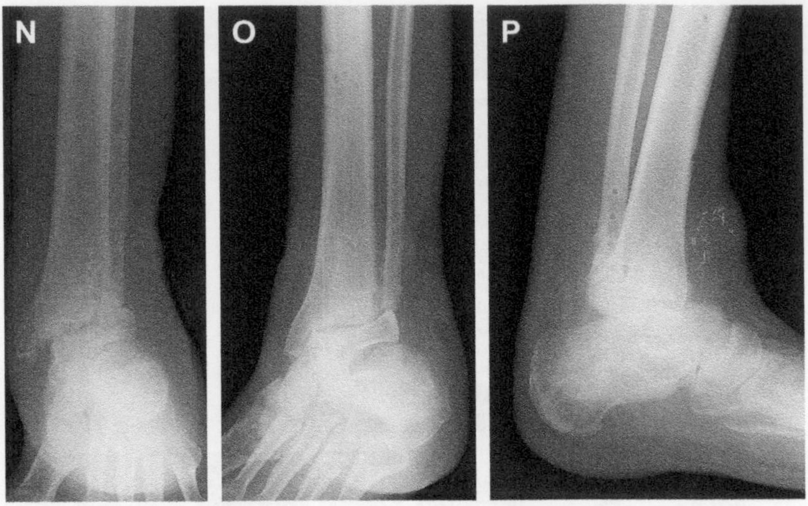

Fig. 2. (*continued*)

of non–weight bearing; and increase the number of office visits in patients who have diabetes and peripheral neuropathy (**Fig. 2**).

Recurrent deformity with or without ulceration

The problems of recurrent Charcot deformity with ulceration, infection, and gross non-unions have led some to advocate amputation in the past. Many investigators have more recently advocated surgical intervention for the failed Charcot reconstruction, however.[2,13,14] Recurrent Charcot deformities are usually the result of a major non-union, isolated joint arthrodesis procedures for multiplane deformities, or exostectomy procedures in the presence of joint instability.

Reports of nonunions for foot and ankle procedures vary in the literature, but increased rates have been implicated in patients undergoing arthrodesis type procedures for CN.[14–20] Several researchers report that nonunions are acceptable in the diabetic patient who has peripheral neuropathy provided that the limb is stable and with an improved alignment when braced and resistant to further skin breakdown while resuming an ambulatory status.[12,21–23] Nonunion can potentially be problematic in this patient population if it leads to mechanical failure of fixation, an unstable limb, further collapse of the deformity making the limb nonbraceable, or infection, however, and additional surgical intervention is required to address these complications.

Shibata and colleagues[12] reported their results on arthrodesis of the ankle for leprotic neuroarthropathy. Twenty-four patients who had arthrodesis of one or both ankles for leprotic neuroarthropathy were followed for an average of 9 years and 5 months. At surgery, after the removal of cartilage, joint debris, and sclerotic bone, the ankle joint was transfixed with an intramedullary nail and staples or Kirschner wires were used to control rotation. Fusion of bone was obtained in 19 of the 26 ankles. Failure to obtain fusion was attributable to postoperative infection in 4 patients, deficiency of the site of arthrodesis in 1 patient, and refracture through the site of fusion in 2 patients. When arthrodesis was successful, additional neuroarthropathic destruction of the midtarsal joint was halted and the preoperative clinical symptoms of dull pain, local warmth, swelling, and instability were relieved.[12]

Schwarz and colleagues[24] retrospectively reported their results of arthrodesis for the treatment of deformities secondary to neuropathic arthropathy to leprosy. Surgery was indicated for acute ongoing instability or recurrent neuropathic bone disintegration and to manage deformity that caused ulceration over bony prominences. All their patients were of Eichenholz stage 2 or 3 at the time of surgery. The following arthrodeses were performed: subtalar (n =16), triple (n = 24), ankle (n = 49), pantalar (n = 11), and other (n = 10). In their study, the primary method of fixation was with a staple, Steinman pin, or combination of the two. These investigators stated that minimal bone grafting was used during their surgical reconstruction and that they achieved deformity correction in 76% of patients, with an overall 88% fusion rate.[24]

Revisional surgery for recurrent deformity correction or nonunions in the neuropathic lower extremity is best managed with eradication of infection if present, joint realignment, and arthrodesis. Often, multiple joints require arthrodesis to achieve the required stability of the extremity for ambulation. Extended joint arthrodesis procedures allow the correction of multiplane deformities to achieve stability while preventing recurrent deformity about the neuropathic lower extremity. The notion of preserving motion by foregoing an extended arthrodesis procedure could lead to a future Charcot event and deformity about an adjacent joint requiring further surgical intervention.

Role of Achilles tendon lengthening

It has been well documented that there are increased vertical forces acting on the feet of diabetic patients with neuropathic ulcerations, many of whom perhaps have an Achilles tendon contracture.[25] An Achilles tendon contracture exacerbates problems associated with diabetic neuropathic osteoarthropathy. The Achilles tendon of the patient who has CN has significantly altered physical properties compared with a normal tendon. Biomechanical test data show that there is a significant difference in ultimate tensile strength and elasticity between tendons of patients who have a Charcot foot and those of non-Charcot controls.[26] A tight Achilles tendon can lead to increased pressure in the plantar hindfoot, midfoot, and forefoot.[27] This alone can cause ulceration or initiate a Charcot process in patients with decreased sensation.[7] An equinus contracture not only increases plantar peak pressures but stresses adjacent joints, frequently causing them to collapse and develop into nonreducible deformities. The rationale for performing a tendo–Achilles tendon lengthening or gastrocnemius recession is to reduce a deformity and prevent further destructive forces across the midtarsus. This procedure is typically performed in adjunct to osseous reconstruction of Charcot "rockerbottom" deformities. Prophylactic Achilles tendon lengthening to prevent ulceration or deformity is controversial. Lengthening the Achilles tendon does decrease the plantar and midfoot pressures acutely, but the long-term effect is still to be determined. Pressures have been shown to increase over time despite the Achilles tendon being lengthened. In addition, the risk for rupture or overlengthening of the Achilles tendon is associated with major complications in this patient population. The complications associated with lengthening the Achilles tendon in the diabetic population arise from overlengthening, iatrogenic rupture of the tendon during the procedure, and late rupture secondary to ambulation with a weakened tendon.

Lengthening of the Achilles tendon has been recommended in healing plantar neuropathic ulceration of the forefoot. Overly aggressive lengthening of an Achilles tendon contracture can result in a complete rupture in the immediate postoperative course or as a late complication, however. Rupture of the Achilles tendon has been reported in 10% of patients after percutaneous tendo–Achilles tendon lengthening.[28] This can be detrimental in patients with a loss of protective sensation in the heel area. An overlengthened Achilles tendon can lead to a calcaneal gait pattern and transfer of lesions or ulcerations to the plantar aspect of the heel. Achilles tendon ruptures in the neuropathic patient can lead to increased edema, hematoma, infection, and even limb loss if not treated acutely. Ankle instability can become apparent, and the surgeon can appreciate unresisted dorsiflexion. In addition, with loss of plantar flexion, the patient is susceptible to heel ulceration and further Charcot processes. The authors have found that salvage of this devastating complication is best achieved with an ankle or tibiotalocalcaneal arthrodesis, because repair of the tendon is not feasible and is not usually recommended in this patient population.

Soft tissue infection and osteomyelitis

Careful preoperative evaluation, timing of surgery, and optimization and treatment of associated comorbidities and underlying risk factors are fundamental to reduce the risks associated with revisional limb salvage surgery. Diabetes mellitus, now the leading cause of CN, is a multisystem disorder that can have a profound effect on the patient's immune system, making him or her susceptible to severe limb-threatening infections, especially when associated with an underlying deformity and previously unsuccessful surgery. Optimal medical control of diabetes and associated comorbidities is crucial before performing "elective" reconstructive foot and ankle surgery.[29] Elevated glycosylated hemoglobin, peripheral vascular disease, malnourishment, decreased collagen synthesis, and impaired cellular proliferation and granulocyte function are a few of the reasons for infection and delayed wound healing in patients who have diabetes.[30]

In the presence of a limb or life-threatening infection after the original Charcot reconstruction, however, the metabolic control and optimization of the diabetic patient are usually initiated at the same time as the urgent or emergent surgery. These complex cases that require medical and surgical management of the underlying infection and osteomyelitis need to be staged, and the timing must be coordinated well in advance with all the medical specialties involved in the patient's care. Before surgery, if an infection is part of the underlying pathologic process, a thorough discussion with the patient should inform him or her regarding the potential for multiple surgical interventions, a prolonged course of treatment, the importance of patient compliance, and the possibility of inability to eradicate the infection.

Conversely, patients may realize at some point that a partial foot or transtibial amputation is their best treatment modality. The authors have found consultations with physical and rehabilitation medicine specialists to be helpful in educating a patient about amputations and prosthesis when the patient is trying to decide between reconstruction–limb salvage and definitive amputation. The surgeon may also need to consider the condition of the contralateral lower extremity before offering a major limb amputation as the best scenario. If the contralateral extremity has poor blood flow, skin breakdown, previous partial pedal amputations, or Charcot deformity, possible limb salvage may be feasible because the likelihood of the patient becoming a bilateral amputee is extremely high.

Appropriate studies should be ordered initially and compared with previous studies if possible to identify the potential for infection or wound healing problems. Laboratory studies may include a complete blood cell count with differential, sedimentation rate, C-reactive protein concentration, blood cultures, albumin level, prealbumin level, chemistry panel, and glycosylated hemoglobin concentration. A serum albumin level greater than 3.5 g/dL is indicative of an adequate nutritional status.[29] In the presence of diminished pulses, noninvasive vascular studies, such arterial Doppler studies with pulsed volume recordings and transcutaneous oxygen pressures or toe pressures, are helpful. Although arterial Doppler readings can be falsely elevated, transcutaneous oxygen pressure measurements can be useful in determining whether local tissue perfusion is sufficient to permit healing. Patients who have a transcutaneous Po_2 value less than 40 mm Hg are poor candidates for reconstructive procedures until it can be improved.[30] Absolute toe pressures, indicative of end-arterial flow, that are greater than 45 mm Hg suggest sufficient blood flow for wound healing.[30]

Appropriate antibiotic selection depends on the types of cultures and the techniques for gathering cultures. Often, patients who are admitted to the hospital for revisional Charcot surgery with infection have been on previous antibiotics. In addition, previous cultures may not have been taken appropriately to identify the primary causative agent. Repeated cultures may be even more difficult, especially when "negative" results are reported and there are clinical signs of infection. In these case scenarios, antibiotics must be stopped for several days and deep intraoperative bone or soft tissue cultures are obtained, along with an appropriate specimen for histopathologic analysis. It is important to include anaerobic cultures in the appropriate transport media because this is commonly overlooked in the treatment of diabetic foot infections. During surgery, if the goal is to obtain a specimen to confirm a deep infection or to direct specific antibiotic therapies, this must be done meticulously. A frozen section or cultures should be taken from the appropriate sites, placed and labeled in the proper container, and sent for pathologic examination immediately. Surgical staging of débridements is helpful in defining viable tissue. At the index procedure, methylene blue is used to visualize nonviable tissue better and all stained tissue is removed. Hardware is removed if it is loosely fixated to bone, and the extremity is stabilized with external fixation devices and pin or wire placement away from the infected surgical site(s).

SUMMARY

In summary, reconstruction of the Charcot foot should eliminate deformity and remove high-pressure areas of the foot and ankle. Most published studies are small, anecdotal, short term, and retrospective. Long-term outcomes, including functional evaluations and quality-of-life studies, are needed. Nonetheless, reconstructive revisional surgery should help to prevent ulceration and infection while resuming an ambulatory status. The reconstructive surgeon must have a thorough preoperative discussion with all patients, and this should include provision of information about lengthy postoperative recovery, the importance of compliance, and potential complications after nonoperative and operative interventions of Charcot surgery and limb salvage. Amputations should also be discussed as an option if all else fails. When complications do occur, the treatment must be individualized to the patient. Adjunctive therapies, including bone grafting, orthobiologics, electrical bone stimulation, and pharmacologic therapy, are crucial to the successful outcome of the patient undergoing revisional Charcot surgery.

This article presented an overview of the most common complications that occur with surgical intervention of the Charcot foot and ankle. Nonsurgical and surgical principles were outlined to assist in the management of revisional Charcot surgery and diabetic limb salvage.

REFERENCES

1. Roukis T, Zgonis T. The management of acute Charcot fracture—dislocations with the Taylor's spatial external fixation system. Clin Podiatr Med Surg 2006;23:467–83.
2. Zgonis T, Roukis TS, Lamm BM. Charcot foot and ankle reconstruction: current thinking and surgical approaches. Clin Podiatr Med Surg 2007;24:505–17.

3. Frykberg RG, Zgonis T, Armstrong DG, et al. Diabetic foot disorders: a clinical practice guideline. J Foot Ankle Surg 2006;45(05):S1–66.
4. Larsen K, Fabrin J, Holstein PE. Incidence and management of ulcers in diabetic Charcot feet. J Wound Care 2001;10(8):323–8.
5. Cooper PS. Application of external fixators for management of Charcot deformities of the foot and ankle. Foot Ankle Clin 2002;7(1):207–54.
6. Stuart M, Morrey B. Diabetic neuropathic ankle arthrodesis. Clin Orthop Relat Res 1990;253:209–11.
7. Garapati R, Weinfeld SB. Complex reconstruction of the diabetic foot and ankle. Am J Surg 2004;187(5A):81S–6S.
8. Hedlund LJ, Maki DD, Griffiths HJ. Calcaneal fractures in diabetic patients. J Diabet Complications 1998;12:81–7.
9. Kathol M, El-Khoury G, Moore T, et al. Calcaneal insufficiency avulsion fractures in patients with diabetes mellitus. Radiology 1991;180(3):725–9.
10. Foltz KD, Fallat LM, Schwartz S. Usefulness of a brief assessment battery for early detection of Charcot foot deformity in patients with diabetes. J Foot Ankle Surg 2004;43(2):87–92.
11. Frykberg RG, Belczyk R. Epidemiology of the Charcot foot. Clin Podiatr Med Surg 2008;25:17–28.
12. Shibata T, Tada K, Hashizume C. The results of arthrodesis of the ankle for leprotic neuroarthropathy. J Bone Joint Surg Am 1990;72(5):749–56.
13. Wang JC, Le AW, Tsukuda RK. A new technique for Charcot's foot reconstruction. J Am Podiatr Med Assoc 2002;92(8):429–36.
14. Saxena A, DiDomenico L, Widtfeldt A, et al. Implantable electrical bone stimulation for arthrodeses of the foot and ankle in high-risk patients: a multicenter study. J Foot Ankle Surg 2005;44(6):450–4.
15. Lau JT, Stamatis ED, Myerson MS, et al. Implantable direct-current bone stimulators in high-risk and revision foot and ankle surgery: a retrospective analysis with outcome assessment. Am J Orthop 2007;36(7):354–7.
16. Hockenbury RT, Gruttadauria M, McKinney I. Use of implantable bone growth stimulation in Charcot ankle arthrodesis. Foot Ankle Int 2007;28(9):971–6.
17. Hanft J, Goggin J, Landsman A, et al. The role of combined magnetic field bone growth stimulation as an adjunct in the treatment of neuroarthropathy/Charcot joint: an expanded pilot study. J Foot Ankle Surg 1998;37(6):510–5.
18. Samilson RL, Sankaran B, Bersani F, et al. Orthopaedic management of neuropathic joints. Arch Surg 1959;78:115–21.
19. Johnson J. Neuropathic fractures and joint injuries: pathogenesis and rationale of prevention and treatment. J Bone Joint Surg Am 1967;49:1–30.
20. Harris JR, Brand PW. Patterns of disintegration of the tarsus in the anaesthetic foot. J Bone Joint Surg Br 1966;48(1):4–16.
21. Pinzur MS, Sostak J. Surgical stabilization of nonplantigrade Charcot arthropathy of the midfoot. Am J Orthop 2007;36(7):361–5.
22. Pinzur MS. The role of ring external fixation in Charcot foot arthropathy. Foot Ankle Clin 2006;11(4):837–47.
23. Pinzur MS. Neutral ring fixation for high-risk nonplantigrade Charcot midfoot deformity. Foot Ankle Int 2007;28(9):961–6.
24. Schwarz R, Macdonald M, Van der Pas M. Results of arthrodesis in neuropathic feet. J Bone Joint Surg Br 2006;88:747–50.
25. Ctercteko G, Dhanendran M, Hutton W, et al. Vertical forces acting on the feet of diabetic patients with neuropathic ulceration. Br J Surg 1981;68:608–14.

26. Grant WP, Foreman EJ, Wilson AS, et al. Evaluation of Young's modulus in Achilles tendons with diabetic neuroarthropathy. J Am Podiatr Med Assoc 2005;95(3): 242–6.
27. Lin S, Lee T, Wapner K. Plantar forefoot ulceration with equinus deformity of the ankle in diabetic patients: the effect of tendo-Achilles lengthening and total contact casting. Orthopaedics 1996;19:465–75.
28. Holstein P, Lohmann M, Bitsch M, et al. Achilles tendon lengthening, the panacea for plantar forefoot ulceration? Diabetes Metab Res Rev 2004;20:37–40.
29. Onzur A, Zgonis T. Closure of major diabetic foot wounds and defects with external fixation. Clin Podiatr Med Surg 2007;24:519–28.
30. Padanilam T, Donley B. High-risk foot and ankle patients. Foot Ankle Clin 2003;8: 149–57.

Current Concepts and Techniques in Foot and Ankle Surgery

The Use of Ilizarov Technique as a Definitive Percutaneous Reduction for Ankle Fractures in Patients Who Have Diabetes Mellitus and Peripheral Vascular Disease

Lawrence A. DiDomenico, DPM, FACFAS[a,*], Damieon Brown, DPM[a], Thomas Zgonis, DPM, FACFAS[b]

KEYWORDS

- Ilizarov external fixation • Diabetes mellitus • Ankle fracture
- Peripheral neuropathy • Peripheral vascular disease

More frequently, trauma surgeons in the United States use external fixation to stabilize lower extremity fractures temporarily until the soft tissue envelopes are prepared for surgery.[1,2] Open reduction internal fixation (ORIF) is then executed after the decrease in soft tissue swelling and when the skin lines are present in the nonvascularly compromised patient.[3] Standard treatment for a similar case would involve a period of non-weight bearing for approximately 6 to 8 weeks, followed by limited protected weight bearing and evidence of radiographic bone healing throughout the postoperative period. In a previous study reported from Sweden,[4] a great deal of emphasis was placed on early weight bearing after ORIF of ankle fractures for patients who did not have diabetes mellitus or dense peripheral neuropathy.

[a] Ohio College of Podiatric Medicine, Ankle and Foot Care Centers, Youngstown, OH, USA
[b] Department of Orthopaedic Surgery, Division of Podiatric Medicine and Surgery, The University of Texas Health Science Center at San Antonio, San Antonio, TX, USA
* Corresponding author.
E-mail address: LD5353@aol.com (L. A. DiDomenico).

Clin Podiatr Med Surg 26 (2009) 141–148
doi:10.1016/j.cpm.2008.09.005

Over the past 5 decades, the prevalence and severity of ankle fractures have increased in individuals.[5] Treatment of ankle fractures among diabetic patients tends to be fraught with increased complication rates, however, and poses unique challenges for the treating physician.[2] Peripheral vascular disease or peripheral neuropathy is presumed to be a contributing factor leading to higher complications in the treatment of ankle fractures.[6] As a result, infection, wound healing problems, nonunions, and loss of fixation tend to be the end result.[7] Low and Tran[8] performed a retrospective review of 10 diabetic patients treated surgically for ankle fractures and noted four wound infections, two of which resulted in transtibial amputation. Based on this study, they concluded that infection was considered a major problem in diabetic patients treated surgically for ankle fractures. There have also been several case-controlled studies reported on surgical treatment of ankle fractures in diabetic patients. Results have shown an overall complication rate of 43%, with the infection rate being 30%.[8–10]

McCormack and Leith[11] performed a review of 26 diabetic patients with displaced malleolar fractures and a cohort group. They noted an overall complication rate of 42% in the diabetic patients compared with no complications in the cohort group. Six of the 19 patients treated surgically developed a deep infection, and 2 patients eventually required an amputation at an unspecified level. The major complication noted in the nonoperative group revealed loss of reduction and malunion. Blotter and colleagues[9] performed a retrospective review of 21 patients who had diabetes and 46 randomly selected patients who did not have diabetes and were treated surgically for ankle fracture and reported a 43% complication rate in the diabetic patients compared with 16% in the nondiabetic group. The complications in this review were noted to be more severe in patients who had diabetes mellitus, including deep infections, and, thereafter, some of the patients required a below-the-knee amputation. In 2000, Flynn and colleagues[12] retrospectively reviewed 25 patients who had diabetes and 73 patients who did not have diabetes and were treated surgically or nonsurgically for closed ankle fracture. This study revealed that diabetic patients were likely to have infection develop 32% of the time compared with 8% of the time in patients who did not have diabetes. They concluded that diabetic patients who were noted to have signs of peripheral vascular disease, neuropathy, severe swelling, or ecchymosis were poor surgical candidates and most prone to infection and complications with their surgery.

Although the aforementioned studies discuss diabetic and nondiabetic patients, they all emphasize that these injuries can have disastrous results, with infection rates ranging from 17% to 50% and amputation rates of 4% to 17%.[7] Peripheral vascular disease, peripheral neuropathy, poor bone quality, poor immune function, and diminished healing potential, coupled with poor compliance, are noted prognostic factors for poor results.[7]

In this article, the authors demonstrate an alternative technique that may be useful in the surgeon's toolbox when dealing with the immunocompromised diabetic patient (peripheral vascular disease or peripheral neuropathy) and the presence of an unstable ankle fracture. The authors recommend that percutaneous reduction with an Ilizarov type circular external fixator can generate a construct that maintains anatomic alignment and simultaneous compression across the fracture site(s) and may allow early and full weight bearing if needed during the postoperative period.

SURGICAL TECHNIQUE

The initial clinical presentation is a valuable predictor of what additional surgical steps might be required. Radiographic examination, along with a CT scan, should be obtained to confirm a diagnosis and determine the severity of pathologic findings (**Fig. 1**).

After obtaining a thorough and complete past medical history, a physical examination is performed. In the physical examination, close attention is noted to the vascular and neurologic status in addition to the integrity of the skin. The presence of peripheral vascular disease can be demonstrated by decreased or absent pedal pulses, presence of skin necrosis, and atrophic skin. These changes should be closely evaluated and further documented by Doppler testing or noninvasive studies. It is for those diabetic patients who present with signs of peripheral vascular disease that this proposed technique is indicated. The overall operative treatment goals in this patient population are to maintain an articular surface, along with the axial alignment and length of the tibia and fibula, and to prevent any further risks for soft tissue complications.

After the initiation of anesthesia, the patient is placed on a fracture table. The entire lower extremity is prepared above the knee. Attention is directed to the posterior/inferior calcaneus, where a transfixion pin is placed medially to laterally through the body of the calcaneus, ensuring avoidance of injury to the neurovascular structures. Subsequent to the placement of the transfixion pin, a Bohler's clamp is attached to the pin and weights are applied for traction to obtain ligamentotaxis. Once ligamentotaxis is accomplished and the fracture is out to length, fluoroscopy is introduced to the surgical site. Based on the fracture type, olive wires are used for reduction and anatomic alignment under fluoroscopy. For example, if there is a trimalleolar fracture, the medial malleolus is reduced and percutaneously fixated, with olive wires being perpendicular to the fracture line. Next, attention is directed toward the fibular fracture. An olive wire is percutaneously placed perpendicular to the fracture line in an anterior-to-posterior direction. Then, another olive wire is placed perpendicular to the posterior-to-anterior direction. If a large posterior malleolus fracture is identified, another olive wire is percutaneously inserted in a posterior-to-anterior direction and perpendicular to the fracture line. If a pilon fracture is present, the same approach is considered, with the addition of adding olive wires perpendicular to the more proximal fracture fragments (**Fig. 2**).

After the fracture reductions and good anatomic alignment with the olive wires, multiple fine wires are used to build a multiplane circular external fixator to construct a secure external fixator block. This multiplane circular construct is built with a fine-wire technique and provides stability for the entire lower extremity. Once the circular ring fixator is mounted, tensioned, and stabilized, the opposed ends of the olive wires opposite the fractures are secured off the stable external fixator block. Next, each of the olive wires (opposite side of the olive) is tensioned to 90 to 110 kg (based on the bone quality) for compression across the fracture lines. The olive wire(s) is then secured to the stable external fixator block. The olive wires that are tensioned off the stable block allow for compression across the fracture line through the olive wires.

The estimated time for bony consolidation is approximately double the time normally estimated for a patient who does not have diabetes mellitus. Prolonged stabilization is essential to prevent neuropathic fractures from progressing into a Charcot deformity. A patient who has diabetic neuropathy and the presence of peripheral vascular disease generally has consolidation at 12 to 16 weeks. After frame removal, the patient then progresses to a walking-assisted device for approximately 4 to 6 weeks and further bracing for up to 12 months. Frequent postoperative visits, along with patient education and close monitoring, are essential to the patient's overall successful outcome.

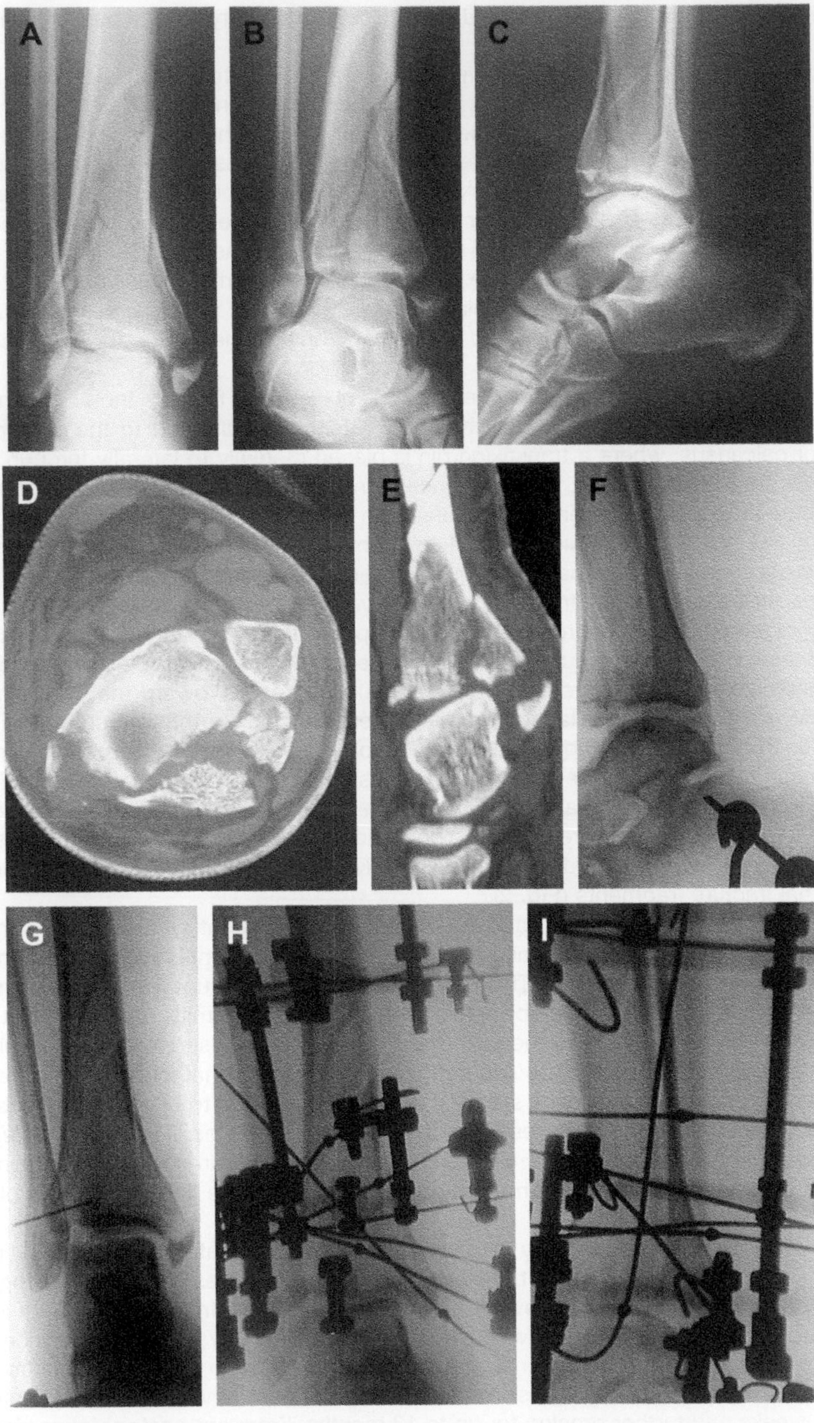
A
B
C
D
E
F
G
H
I

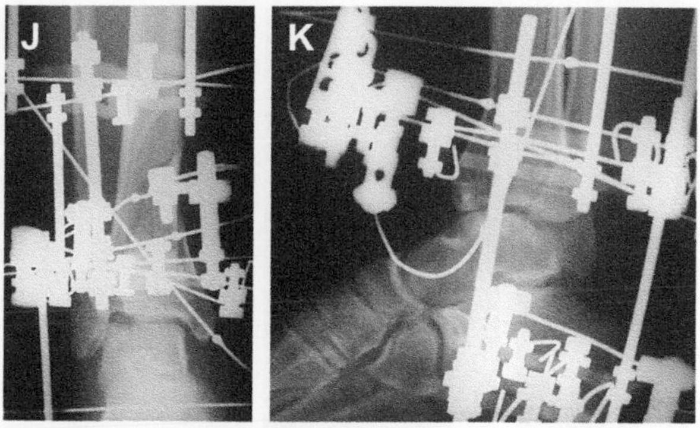

Fig. 1. (*continued*)

DISCUSSION

The use of external fixation has gained a popular role in staged protocols as a primary tool for reduction and preliminary fixation until soft tissue consolidation makes internal fixation feasible.[13] Limited literature is currently available to demonstrate the use of external fixation for acute ankle fracture repair in the vascularly compromised patient with an emphasis on early weight bearing and permanent fixation and on reducing the chance of a second operation to implant internal hardware.

Sound principles and techniques of external fixation are necessary to minimize postoperative complications in diabetic patients who have vascular disease and ankle fractures. Timing of surgery, soft tissue monitoring, proper surgical techniques, and an understanding of the bone healing process in a patient who has dense peripheral diabetic neuropathy are paramount to the patient's long term successful outcome.

Finally, the authors want to emphasize that this particular technique may be applied in a selective group of patients, including but not limited to diabetic patients with the presence of an unstable ankle fracture and peripheral vascular disease.

Fig. 1. Preoperative anterior-posterior (*A*), medial oblique (*B*), and lateral (*C*) radiographic views show an intra-articular distal tibial fracture in a vascularly compromised diabetic patient. (*D, E*) CT scan was ordered at the initial presentation, showing the extent and severity of the fracture. Intraoperative views demonstrate the Bohler's clamp in the calcaneus (*F*) with weight distraction off a fracture table aligning and reducing the fractures by means of ligamentotaxis (*G*). In *G*, note the placement of the small needles as landmarks for the fracture location. Immediate anterior-posterior (*H*) and lateral (*I*) postoperative films show fracture repair by means of the use of multiple percutaneous tensioned olive wires attached to a multiplane circular external fixator. Postoperative anterior-posterior (*J*) and lateral (*K*) views at 5 weeks. The fixator was removed at 12 weeks.

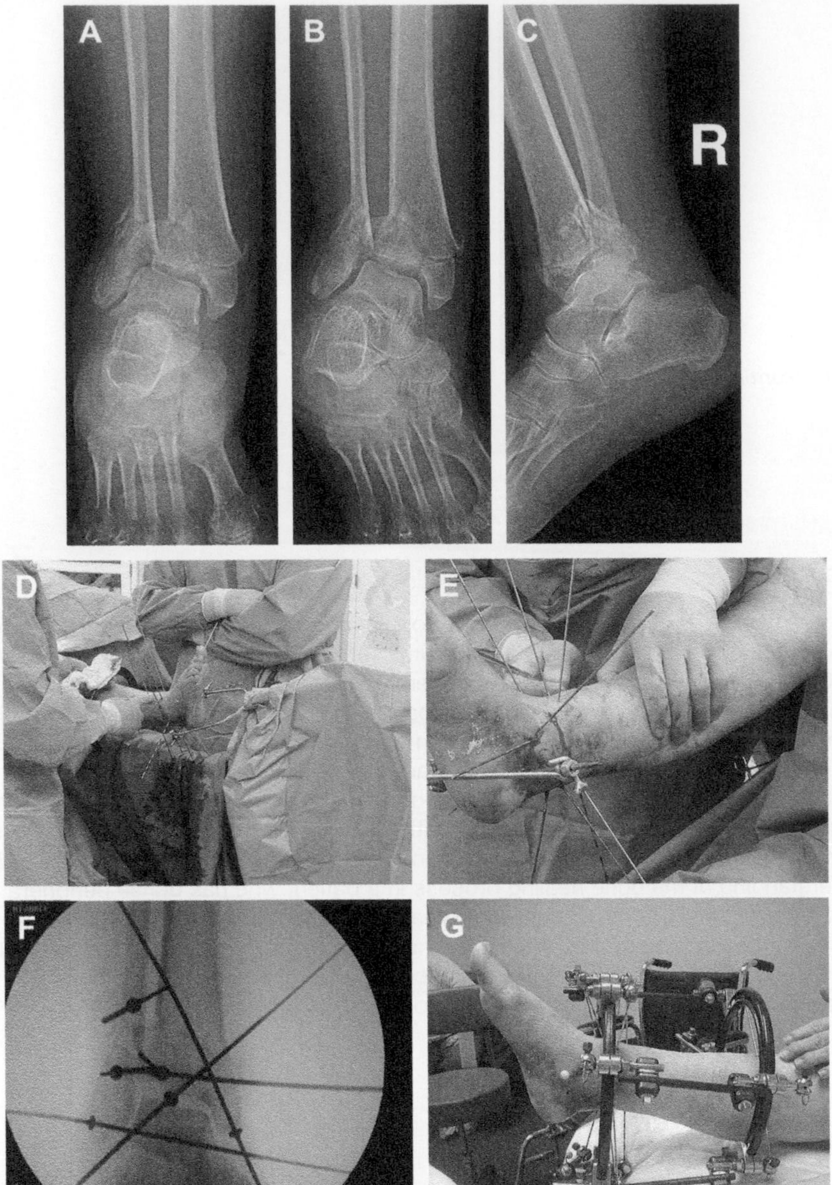

Fig. 2. Preoperative anterior-posterior (*A*), medial oblique (*B*), and lateral (*C*) radiographic views show an intra-articular trimalleolar ankle fracture in a vascularly compromised diabetic patient. (*D*) Intraoperative views demonstrate the Bohler's clamp in the calcaneus with weight distraction off a fracture table aligning and reducing the fractures by means of ligamentotaxis. (*E*) Reduction olive wires are shown in place across the fracture fragments. (*F*) Intraoperative view shows anatomic reduction and ankle joint preservation with the use of multiple percutaneous tensioned olive wires. (*G*) Clinical picture at 3 weeks after surgery. The fixator was removed at 12 weeks. (*H–J*) Clinical views of dorsiflexion and plantarflexion at 6 months.

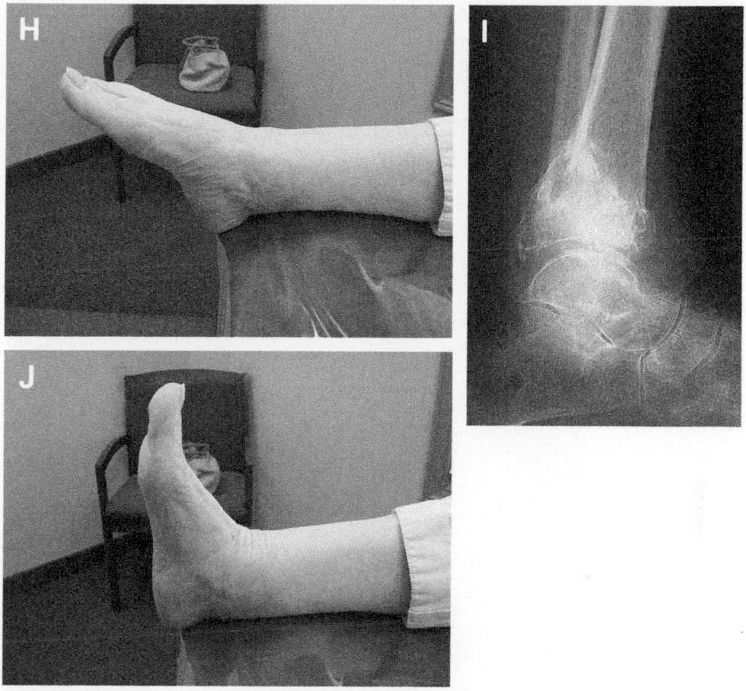

Fig. 2. (*continued*)

REFERENCES

1. Seibert FJ, Fankhauser F, Elliott B, et al. External fixation in trauma of the foot and ankle. Clin Podiatr Med Surg 2003;20(1):159–80.
2. Jones KB, Maiers-Yelden KA, Marsh JL, et al. Ankle fractures in patients with diabetes mellitus. J Bone Joint Surg Br 2005;87(4):489–95.
3. Thordarson DB. Ankle fractures in diabetics. Techniques In Foot and Ankle Surgery 2004;3(3):192–7.
4. Ahl T, Dalén N, Holmberg S, et al. Early weight bearing of displaced ankle fractures. Acta Orthop Scand 1987;58:535–8.
5. Makwana NK, Bhowal B, Harper WM, et al. Conservative versus operative treatment for displaced ankle fracture in patients over 55 years of age. A prospective randomized study. J Bone Joint Surg Br 2001;83(4):525–9.
6. Jani MM, Ricci WM, Borrelli J, et al. A protocol for treatment of unstable ankle fractures using transarticular fixation in patients with diabetes mellitus and loss of protective sensibility. Foot Ankle Int 2003;24(11):838–44.
7. White CB, Turner NS, Lee GC, et al. Open ankle fractures in patients with diabetes mellitus. Clin Orthop Relat Res 2003;414:37–44.
8. Low CK, Tan SK. Infection in the diabetic patients with ankle fractures. Ann Acad Med Singapore 1995;24:353–5.
9. Blotter RH, Connolly E, Wasan A, et al. Acute complications in the operative treatment of isolated ankle fractures in patients with diabetes mellitus. Foot Ankle Int 1999;20:687–94.
10. Kristiansen B. Results of surgical treatment of malleolar fractures in patients with diabetes mellitus. Dan Med Bull 1983;30:272–4.

11. McCormack RG, Leith JM. Ankle fractures in diabetics: complications of surgical management. J Bone Joint Surg Br 1998;80:689–92.
12. Flynn JM, Rodriguez-del Rio F, Piza PA. Closed ankle fractures in the diabetic patient. Foot Ankle Int 2000;21:311–9.
13. Rammelt S, Endres T, Grass R, et al. The role of external fixation in acute ankle trauma. Foot Ankle Clin 2004;9(3):455–74.

Pan–Metatarsophalangeal Joint Arthrodesis for the Severe Rheumatoid Forefoot Deformity

Luke C. Jeffries, DPM, AACFAS[a], Roberto H. Rodriguez, DPM, AACFAS[a], John J. Stapleton, DPM, AACFAS[b,c], Thomas Zgonis, DPM, FACFAS[a,*]

KEYWORDS

- Metatarsophalangeal joint arthrodesis • Rheumatoid foot
- Rheumatoid arthritis • Forefoot deformity

EPIDEMIOLOGY AND PATHOPHYSIOLOGY OF RHEUMATOID ARTHRITIS

Affecting approximately 1% of the global population, rheumatoid arthritis (RA) is the most common form of systemic autoimmune inflammatory arthritis. The incidence of the disease is fairly constant across ethnicities, with only some variation noted among certain native American tribes demonstrating an incidence more than double that of the general population.[1,2] RA preferentially affects women over men by a ratio of 2:1 to 4:1. The prevalence of RA increases with age, affecting mostly patients in the sixth and seventh decades of life.[3]

RA commonly affects the joints of the foot and ankle, limiting the patient's ambulatory status. Forefoot deformities are slightly more prevalent than rearfoot and ankle deformities in the population of patients who have RA. The foot is the first site affected in approximately 16% to 19% of reported RA cases. Initial symptoms typically persist between 85% and 94% of the time when the foot and ankle are affected. Twenty-one percent of patients who have RA develop pedal abnormalities associated with the disease process within the first year, with 53% of patients demonstrating symptomatic foot deformity by the third year. Nearly 100% of these patients develop foot deformities within 10 years of disease onset.[4–7]

Despite considerable effort, the underlying cause of RA remains unclear. Nevertheless, the three leading causative contenders for RA are genetic, infectious, and

[a] Division of Podiatric Medicine and Surgery, Department of Orthopaedic Surgery, The University of Texas Health Science Center at San Antonio, 7703 Floyd Curl Drive, MCS 7776, San Antonio, TX 78229, USA
[b] Foot and Ankle Surgery, VSAS, Orthopaedics, Allentown, PA, USA
[c] Penn State College of Medicine, Hershey, PA, USA
* Corresponding author.
E-mail address: zgonis@uthscsa.edu (T. Zgonis).

Clin Podiatr Med Surg 26 (2009) 149–157
doi:10.1016/j.cpm.2008.09.006
podiatric.theclinics.com
0891-8422/08/$ – see front matter

immunologic. Together or separately, these three insults are responsible for this debilitating disease. In addition, there seems to be a clear genetic component to RA, with recent monozygotic twin studies showing a concordance rate of 30% to 50%.[8] RA is strongly associated with class II histocompatibility complex and the human lymphocyte antigen DR4 cell surface marker.[8] Infectious agents have also been identified as possible causes in the development of RA. Furthermore, the discovery of the rheumatoid factor has implicated immunologically mediated insults as a principal cause of RA. The inflammatory response manifested in RA is found to be caused by the interaction between antigens, antibodies, complement, and immune pathways formed by this rheumatoid factor.[8]

DIAGNOSIS AND CLINICAL PRESENTATION

In 1987, the American Rheumatism Association (ARA) developed a classification to clinically diagnose RA based on seven factors:[9] morning stiffness, arthritis of three or more joints, arthritis of hand joints, symmetric arthritis, rheumatoid nodules, positive serum rheumatoid factor, and radiographic findings that are recognized by the ARA. At least four of these seven findings must be present for at least 6 weeks to make the diagnosis of RA.[9]

The most notable clinical findings include hallux valgus deformities, lateral deviation of the lesser digits, rigid digital deformities, lesser metatarsophalangeal joint (MTPJ) dislocations, rheumatoid nodules, and soft tissue ulcerations. Often, metatarsalgia is the chief complaint as metatarsal heads become more prominent on the plantar aspect of the foot secondary to joint dislocation in combination with fat pad atrophy or displacement. As a result, increased vertical and shear plantar forces to the forefoot result in plantar callosities, bursa formation, rheumatoid nodules, and even ulceration. The gait cycle of patients who have RA with forefoot deformities often demonstrates a decreased stride length with minimal or absent heel strike and limited motion at the first MTPJ.

The extra-articular findings associated with RA include rheumatoid nodules, synovitis, tendonitis, fasciitis, neuritis, vasculitis, pulmonary fibrosis, and cardiac complications. Although the disease is systemic and profound extra-articular findings are common, the primary pathologic finding is represented by the inflammatory and hypertrophic progression of the synovium. The synovium allows pannus to penetrate through its synovial environment as it swells and proliferates. The chronic inflammatory response of leukocyte migration and proteolytic enzymes within the pannus then leads to laxity of the joint capsule and destruction of its surrounding cartilaginous and periarticular bone.[10]

Radiographic findings commonly seen in RA include diffuse intra-articular joint erosions, generalized osteopenia, MTPJ subluxations or dislocations, hallux deformities, and lesser toe deformities. The mixture of chronic inflammation, soft tissue attenuation, and erosive osseous changes leads to the multiple deformities that characterize the rheumatoid foot.

SURGICAL HISTORY OF RHEUMATOID FOREFOOT DEFORMITIES

The pan–metatarsal head resection is the most common forefoot reconstructive surgery offered to patients who have rheumatoid MTPJ and digital deformities. This procedure was originally publicized by Hoffman[11] in 1912, who described the resection of all metatarsal heads with a single curved plantar transverse incision proximal to the MTPJs. The main purpose of this procedure was to relieve forefoot pain by removing the prominent metatarsal heads at the plantar surface of the foot. The incision allowed direct exposure of the metatarsal heads, while removing any plantar lesions or bursae, in addition to facilitating the relocation of the displaced fat pad. This type of surgical approach provides little stability, however, with shortening and dislocation of the digits.

In 1951, Larmon[12] described the three dorsal linear incisional approach for pan-metatarsal head resections. Some disadvantages of this technique include a limited surgical exposure to the metatarsal heads associated with severe dorsal MTPJ subluxations or dislocations. As a result, modifications have been made depending on the number of digital or metatarsal head corrections required and the amount of exposure needed for deformity correction. Five dorsal longitudinal incisions and a lazy "S" incision have also been used as modifications for the surgical treatment of the painful rheumatoid forefoot deformity.[13] Careful incision planning and atraumatic handling of the soft tissues is important with multiple incisions to limit neurovascular injury and soft tissue necrosis.

In 1959, Fowler[14] described a dorsal and plantar approach to the forefoot reconstruction of the rheumatoid foot. He recommended a dorsal transverse incision with proximal extensions along the first and fifth metatarsal shafts in addition to a plantar approach with two converging semielliptic incisions encompassing the MTPJs. Through this approach, the base of the proximal phalanges and the metatarsal heads were removed, with relocation of the plantar fat pad on closure.[14] In 1960, Clayton[15] advocated a straight transverse dorsal approach when performing MTPJ arthroplasties, with extensor tenotomies and interposition of the plantar plates.

Correction of the sagittal and transverse plane lesser toe deformities in rheumatoid forefoot reconstruction is commonly performed in conjunction with metatarsal head resections. Sagittal plane lesser digital corrections are mainly approached with proximal interphalangeal joint (PIPJ) arthroplasty, implant arthroplasty, or PIPJ arthrodesis procedures. The surgical procedure of choice remains at the surgeon's discretion, with no firm consensus in the scientific literature. Creating digital stability through arthrodesis procedures reduces recurrence rates and provides a rigid lever arm during ambulation, however. Steinmann pins have been used to maintain stability for arthrodesis or arthroplasty procedures. In addition, the duration the fixation is retained is longer when an arthrodesis is desired. Osteopenia is a problem, and larger diameter wires are often needed and usually are extended across the tarsometatarsal joint for further stability. Conversely, transverse plane lesser digital corrections are usually obtained through correction and relocation at the related MTPJ.

Hoffman[11] advocated addressing first MTPJ pathologic findings through resection of the metatarsal head in conjunction with lesser metatarsal head resections. More recently, variations have included resectional arthroplasty by excising the base of the proximal phalanx with or without soft tissue interposition (Keller arthroplasty), silastic or metallic implant arthroplasty, and arthrodesis of the first MTPJ.[16] Each of these procedures can be used during forefoot reconstruction of the rheumatoid foot. Although the Keller arthroplasty decreases pain along the first MTPJ and allows acute correction, the instability along the first ray may contribute to transfer metatarsalgia and plantar callosities at the adjacent lesser rays, a problem that is often the major reason for the patient to consider forefoot reconstruction in the first place. Implant arthroplasty may be a viable alternative over resection arthroplasty or arthrodesis in an older rheumatoid patient who is less active. High rates of implant failure, osteophyte formation, and osteolysis have led many to be cautious with this procedure, however. Because of its predictability and generally favorable outcome, first MTPJ arthrodesis has recently become a popular procedure. Weight-bearing capacity at the surgical site is greater in patients who underwent arthrodesis procedures versus those who underwent arthroplasty of the first MTPJ. Successful first MTPJ arthrodesis adds stability to the medial column of the foot and compares favorably with arthroplasty in terms of pain relief and patient satisfaction. In addition, arthrodesis of the first MTPJ addresses complaints of metatarsalgia while preventing postoperative transfer lesions. Arthrodesis can also be used to revise unsuccessful surgical outcomes involving the first ray among patients who have RA. Fixation is patient dependent but typically involves the use of Steinmann pins, screws, or plate fixation depending on the inherent quality of the bone.

PAN–METATARSOPHALANGEAL JOINT ARTHRODESIS FOR THE RHEUMATOID FOREFOOT DEFORMITY

The rheumatoid forefoot usually presents with a mild or moderate hallux valgus deformity and concomitant lesser toe contracture without significant joint deformities and metatarsalgia or with the presence of severe joint deformities, dislocations and unstable toe deformities, and painful metatarsalgia. Mild deformities with good bone density can be corrected with a bunionectomy or first metatarsal osteotomy, lesser metatarsal osteotomies, and correction of the lesser digits. Moderate and severe deformities that involve joint erosions, dislocations, soft tissue laxity, transverse plane deformities, and generalized osteopenia are typically managed with arthrodesis or resection arthroplasty hallux MTPJ, resection of the lesser metatarsal heads, and correction of the lesser digits. Within a certain period, however, the recurrence of deformities is likely to occur secondary to soft tissue laxity and ligamentous instability. Recurrent deformities after a previous pan–metatarsal head resection are often difficult to revise because of the significant previous bone resections and voids, thus minimizing the surgical options for revisional surgery. For this reason, the rationale of performing pan–metatarsophalangeal joint (PMTPJ) arthrodesis is to provide long-lasting deformity correction and pain relief while preventing further joint instability. In addition, if revisional surgery needs to be performed, the arthrodesis site(s) can be converted to interpositional arthroplasties if needed.

SURGICAL TECHNIQUE

After initiation of anesthesia, a well-padded thigh tourniquet is placed on the patient's extremity. The procedure is performed with the use of a tourniquet to minimize intraoperative bleeding and decrease the risk for postoperative edema while facilitating visualization of the anatomy during surgical dissection. The authors prefer the five dorsal incisional approach that extends into the distal aspect of the digits when possible (**Fig. 1**). If fragility of the skin or narrow skin bridges could compromise tissue viability, however, the three dorsal linear incisional approach may be used. The decision on skin incisions usually depends on the degree of deformity with the integrity of the skin. Caution should be used with transverse dorsal and plantar incisions with this technique because of the severely contracted dorsal soft tissues. Although, these incisions may be preferable for metatarsal head resections, they are not favorable for lesser MTPJ arthrodesis, which does not result in much shortening of the metatarsal.

The first MTPJ is approached through a 6- to 7-cm dorsal medial longitudinal incision adjacent to the extensor hallucis longus tendon. The incision is deepened directly to bone just medial to the extensor hallucis longus tendon, exposing the MPTJ. Often, the collateral ligaments may be transected and plantar adhesions released with a curved periosteal elevator to expose the joint surfaces adequately. The joint is then prepared for arthrodesis by removing all the joint synovium and remaining articular cartilaginous surfaces. The joint can be prepared with a sagittal saw, osteotome, curette, or ball and socket reamer, because this portion of the procedure is surgeon dependent. Despite the method used for joint preparation, the contour of the joint should be maintained and shortening should be minimized to facilitate appropriate positioning of the hallux. Alignment of the hallux is paramount for a successful outcome and cannot be overlooked. The hallux is often positioned in relation to the floor or a weight-bearing surface as opposed to the alignment of the first metatarsal. Slight dorsiflexion is preferable by simulating a weight-bearing surface to determine the appropriate amount of dorsiflexion desired. Often, the first intermetatarsal angle needs to be reduced, and this can be accomplished with manual medial-to-lateral compression of the forefoot while the hallux is positioned. In addition, the medial and lateral nail folds are used as landmarks to obtain positioning of the hallux in the frontal plane to prevent oversupination or pronation. It is preferable to stabilize the arthrodesis with crossed Steinmann pins whether they are to be used for definitive or temporary fixation before the placement of plates and screws. Intraoperative C-arm imaging is recommended throughout the entire procedure to determine the alignment of the entire forefoot reconstruction. The capsular and subcutaneous tissues are then approximated with absorbable sutures, but skin closure is usually performed at the end of the entire surgical procedure.

After this initial step, attention is then directed to the second through fourth lesser MTPJs and PIPJs, where dorsal longitudinal incisions are made along the MTPJs extending distally into a "lazy S" or serpentine shape when approaching the PIPJs. The incisions along the MTPJs are spaced approximately 1 cm apart. Each incision is carried down to the level of the extensor digitorum tendon, which is tenotomized at the level of the related PIPJ. The medial and collateral ligaments of the PIPJ are then transected, exposing the head of the proximal phalanx and the base of the middle phalanx. The extensor digitorum tendon is then grasped and retracted proximally as the extensor hood apparatus is released with tenotomy scissors proximal to the level of the MTPJ. This technique facilitates exposure of the dislocated joint while minimizing soft tissue dissection medial and lateral to the metatarsal head. Once the MTPJ is identified, an aggressive capsulotomy without tenorrhaphy is performed to expose the joint while simultaneously resecting the joint synovitis. The PIPJs are prepared for arthrodesis through planar joint resection with a sagittal saw. Attention to limited straight linear bone cuts is paramount to prevent future toe irritation. Joint preparation of the lesser MTPJs is then performed. First, any dorsal osteophytes are removed with a small rongeur, and if a ball and socket contour is still present, the remaining articular surfaces can be removed with the same instrumentation. If significant deformity or joint erosions are present, joint resection with a sagittal saw or with small ball and socket reamers is performed. The metatarsal head is excised in a linear direction from a dorsal-to-plantar orientation. It is imperative that the osteotomy not be angulated, as is typically performed with a pan–metatarsal head resection. The toe is then positioned, and the articular surface to the base of the proximal phalanx is removed with a sagittal saw in a reciprocating manner to preserve as much length and contour as possible to the toe. It is also important to note that a simultaneous plantar metatarsal condylectomy is performed at the time of the cartilage resection of the lesser MTPJs to prevent future metatarsalgia. This is done with the use of a curved periosteal elevator and a small osteotome. A pilot hole is then centrally fashioned to the medullary canal of the metatarsal and the proximal phalanx. A Steinman pin is then driven anterograde from the base of the middle phalanx out to the distal aspect of the toe and retrograded across the PIPJ and MTPJ while the toe is anatomically aligned. The position should be checked in relation to the weight-bearing surface and in conjunction with the first MTPJ to form an evenly distributed plane. Small

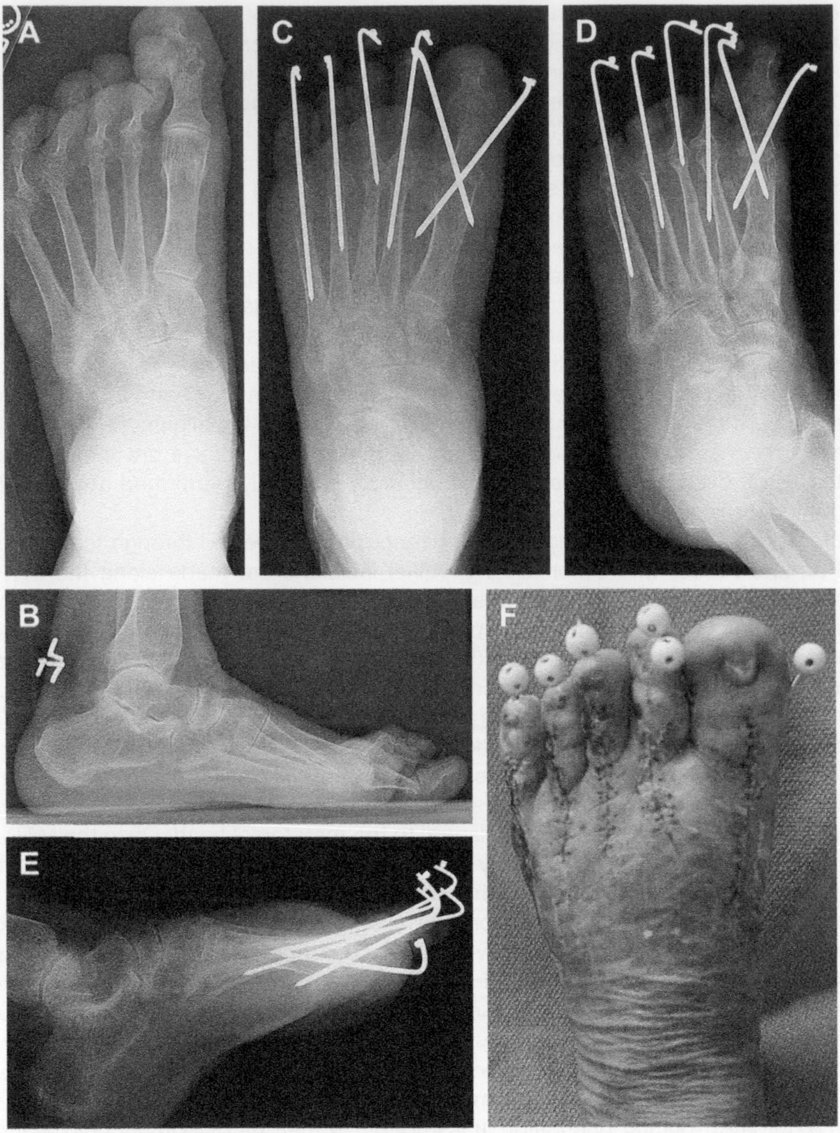

Fig. 1. Anterior-posterior (*A*) and lateral (*B*) preoperative radiographs show the severe rheumatoid forefoot deformity. A patient presented with severe dorsal dislocations of the digits at the MTPJs along with plantar rheumatoid nodules and callosities. The patient was taking prednisone and methotrexate for her RA. Radiographic (*C–E*) and clinical (*F*) views of the reconstructed rheumatoid foot with PMTPJ arthrodesis at 4 weeks after surgery. All wires were removed at 6 weeks after surgery. Final radiographic (*G, H*) and clinical (*I, J*) views at 1 year of follow-up. Note the anatomic alignment of the digits and the absence of any plantar forefoot lesions or ulcerations.

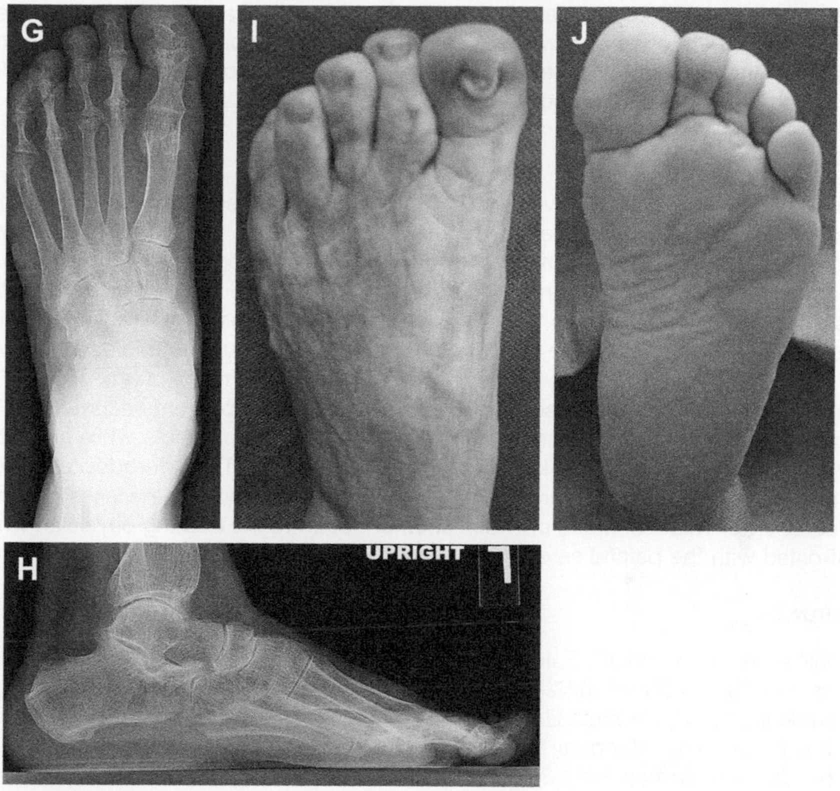

Fig. 1. (*continued*)

gaping at the arthrodesis sites can be augmented with autogenous or allogenic bone grafting if needed. The capsular and subcutaneous tissues are then approximated with absorbable sutures, but skin closure is usually performed at the end of the entire surgical procedure.

Attention is then directed to the fifth ray, where an obliquely oriented elliptic incision is made from a distal-medial to lateral-proximal direction over the fifth PIPJ, with a proximal extension along the fifth MTPJ in a Z-shaped fashion. Both joints are exposed as previously described, and a fifth PIPJ arthroplasty is followed by a fifth partial metatarsal head resection or MTPJ arthrodesis in the manner described for the other lesser rays. The authors favor the latter technique to ensure the favorable long-term outcomes associated with the stability imparted by arthrodesis. A pilot hole is then centrally fashioned to the medullary canal of the metatarsal and the proximal phalanx. A Steinman pin is driven anterograde from the base of the middle phalanx out to the distal aspect of the toe and then retrograded across the PIPJ and MTPJ while the toe is anatomically aligned. Final positioning of the entire forefoot should be checked by means of intraoperative imaging in relation to the weight-bearing surface and in conjunction with the first MTPJ. Skin closure is then performed, and the tourniquet is deflated. Signs of ischemia or severe hematoma are closely monitored at the end of the procedure.

After surgery, the patient is kept non–weight bearing for approximately 6 to 8 weeks and is allowed to weight bear partially with an offloading device after radiographic evidence of bone healing and removal of the wire fixation. In cases in which the patient cannot tolerate crutches or a walker secondary to rheumatoid manifestations of the upper extremity, a surgical shoe with a wedge to offload the forefoot is recommended and weight bearing is permitted through the heel only.

DISCUSSION

Numerous studies seem to favor first MTPJ arthrodesis over joint resection arthroplasty.[17–20] Invariably, the patients who have undergone the arthrodesis procedures report superior long-term cosmetic and functional results compared with the Mayo-Keller cohort.[2,21–23] Implant arthroplasty of the first MTPJ is described and supported by some researchers. Implants, however, are associated with considerable morbidity, including foreign body reaction, bony resorption, implant failure, and infection. It was the authors' intention to extend the well-documented benefits of the first MTPJ arthrodesis to that of the lesser MTPJs.[24] In an effort to prevent recurrent MTPJ deformities, care must be taken to maintain the metatarsal parabola while appropriately positioning the hallux and lesser toes. The proposed PMTPJ arthrodesis obviates the need for aggressive metatarsal head resection, while stabilizing the lesser digits at the same time. This technique provides another option to the treating physician when confronted with the painful severe rheumatoid forefoot deformity.

REFERENCES

1. Silman AJ, Pearson JE. Epidemiology and genetics of rheumatoid arthritis. Arthritis Res 2002;4(Suppl 3):S265–72.
2. Kadenbande S, Debnath U, Kharana A, et al. Rheumatoid forefoot reconstruction: first metatarsophalangeal fusion and excision arthroplasty of lesser metatarsal heads. Acta Orthop Belg 2007;73(1):88–95.
3. Felson DT. Epidemiology of the rheumatic diseases. In: Koopman WJ, editor. Arthritis and allied conditions: a textbook of rheumatology. 13th edition. Baltimore: Williams and Wilkins; 1997. p. 6.
4. Jaakkola JI, Mann RA. A review of rheumatoid arthritis affecting the foot and ankle. Foot Ankle Int 2004;25(12):866–74.
5. Wilder RL. Rheumatoid arthritis. Epidemiology, pathology and pathogenesis. In: Schumacher H, Klippel J, Koopman W, editors. Primer on the rheumatic diseases. 11th edition. Georgia: The Arthritis Foundation; 1997. p. 155-60.
6. Firestein GS, Paine MM, Littman BH. Gene expression (collagenase, tissue inhibitor of metalloproteinases, complement, and HLA-DR) in rheumatoid arthritis and osteoarthritis synovium. Quantitative analysis and effect of intraarticular corticosteroids. Arthritis Rheum 1991;34(9):1094–105.
7. Lawrence RC, Hochberg MC, Kelsy JL. Estimates of the prevalence of selected arthritic and musculoskeletal diseases in the United States. J Rheumatol 1989; 16(4):427–41.
8. Winchester R. The molecular basis of susceptibility to rheumatoid arthritis. Adv Immunol 1994;56:389–466.
9. Arnett FC, Edworthy SM, Bloch DA, et al. The American Rheumatism Association 1987 revised criteria for the classification of rheumatoid arthritis. Arthritis Rheum 1988;31(3):315–24.
10. Harris ED Jr. Rheumatoid arthritis. Pathophysiology and implications for therapy. N Engl J Med 1990;322(18):1277–89.
11. Hoffman P. An operation for severe grades of contracted or clawed toes. J Orthop Surg 1912;9:441–9.

12. Larmon WA. Surgical treatment of deformities of rheumatoid arthritis of the forefoot and toes. Bull. Borthwestern Univ Med School 1951;25:39–42.
13. Brodie JT, Kile TA. The foot in rheumatoid arthritis. In: Bulstrode CJK, Buckwalter J, Carr A, Fairbank J, Marsh L, editors. Oxford textbook of orthopedics and trauma. New York: Oxford University Press; 2002.
14. Fowler AW. A method of forefoot reconstruction. J Bone Joint Surg Br 1959;41: 507–13.
15. Clayton ML. Surgery of the forefoot in rheumatoid arthritis. Clin Orthop 1960;16: 136–40.
16. Keller WL. The surgical treatment of bunions and hallux valgus. New York Med J 1904;80:741–2.
17. Farrow SJ, Kingsley GH, Scott DL. Interventions for foot disease in rheumatoid arthritis: a systematic review. Arthritis Rheum 2005;53(4):593–602.
18. Petrov O, Pfeifer M, Flood M, et al. Recurrent plantar ulceration following pan metatarsal head resection. J Foot Ankle Surg 1996;35(6):573–7.
19. Beuchamp CG, Kirby T, Rudge SR, et al. Fusion of the first metatarsophalangeal joint in forefoot arthroplasty. Clin Orthop Relat Res 1984;190:249–53.
20. Henry AP, Waugh W, Wood H. The use of footprints in assessing the results of operations for hallux valgus. A comparison of Keller's operation and arthrodesis. J Bone Joint Surg Br 1975;57(4):478–81.
21. Coughlin MJ. Rheumatoid forefoot reconstruction. A long-term follow-up study. J Bone Joint Surg Am 2000;82(3):322–41.
22. Mulcahy D, Daniels TR, Lau JT, et al. Rheumatoid forefoot deformity: a comparison study of 2 functional methods of reconstruction. J Rheumatol 2003;30(7): 1440–50.
23. Hughes J, Grace D, Clark P, et al. Metatarsal head excision for rheumatoid arthritis. 4-year follow-up of 68 feet with and without hallux fusion. Acta Orthop Scand 1991;62(1):63–6.
24. Karlock LG. Second metatarsophalangeal joint fusion: a new technique for crossover hammertoe deformity. A preliminary report. J Foot Ankle Surg 2003;42(4): 178–82.

Index

Note: Page numbers of article titles are in **boldface** type.

Clin Podiatr Med Surg 26 (2009) 159–168
doi:10.1016/S0891-8422(08)00106-7

H

I

J

K

Printed and bound by CPI Group (UK) Ltd, Croydon, CR0 4YY
03/10/2024
01040465-0017